The Current Perspectives on Coronary Artery Bypass Grafting

Edited by Takashi Murashita

Published in London, United Kingdom

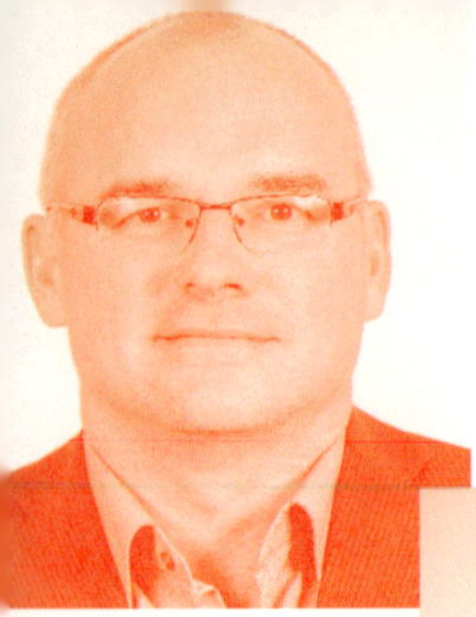
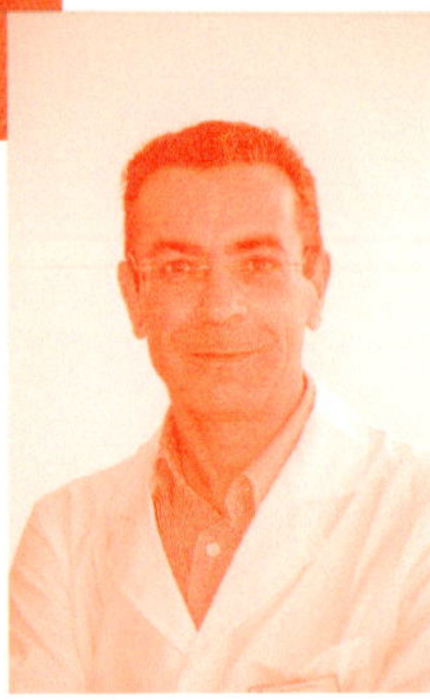
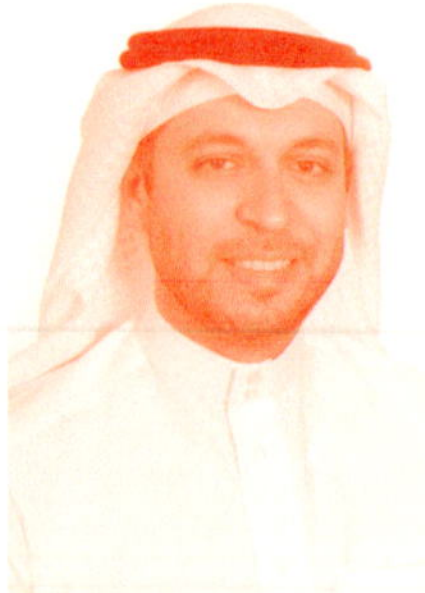
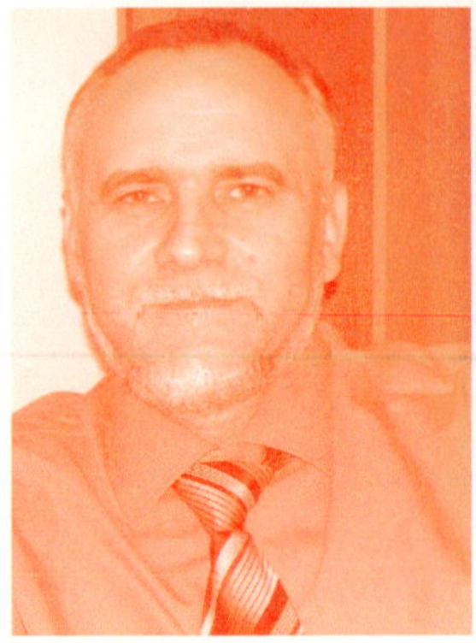
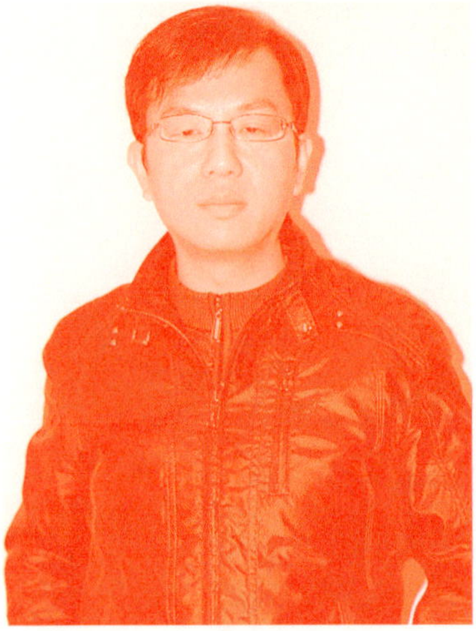
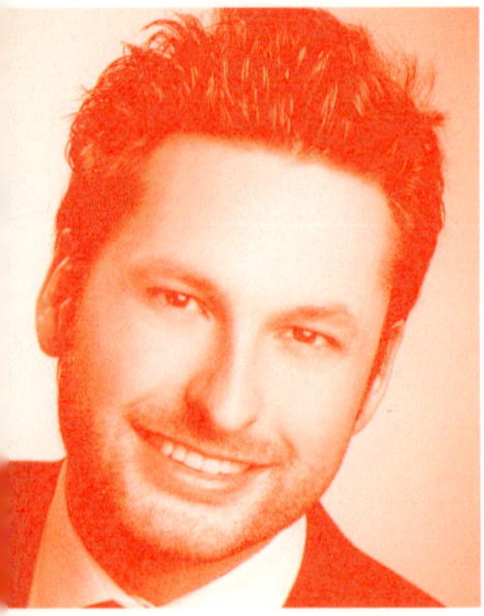
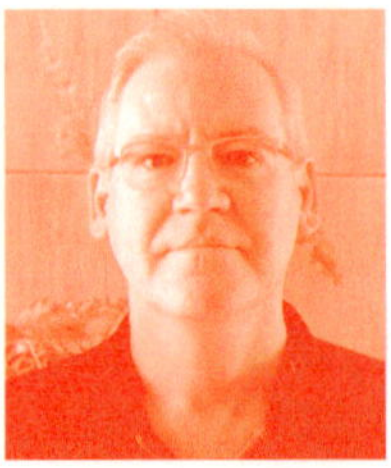

IntechOpen

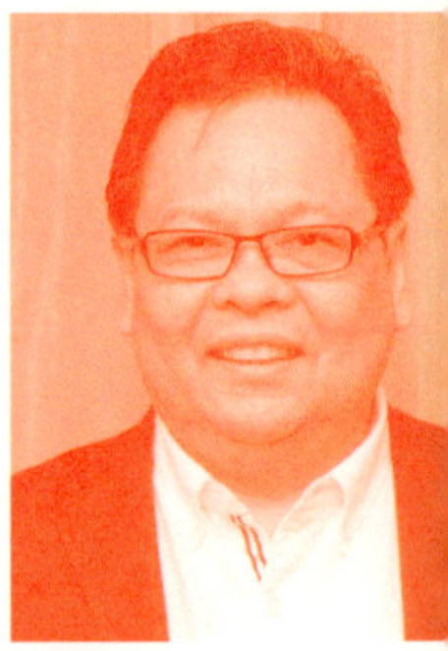
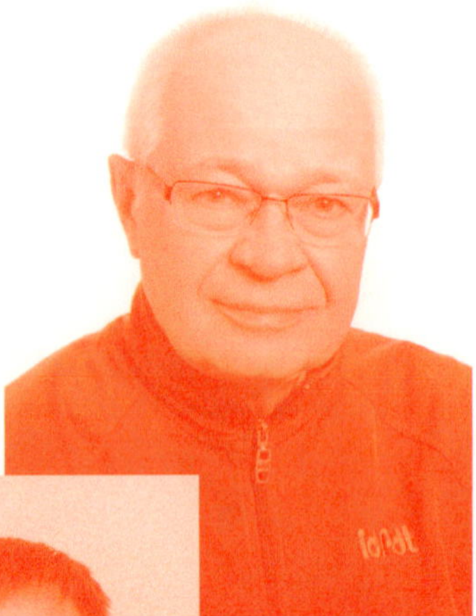
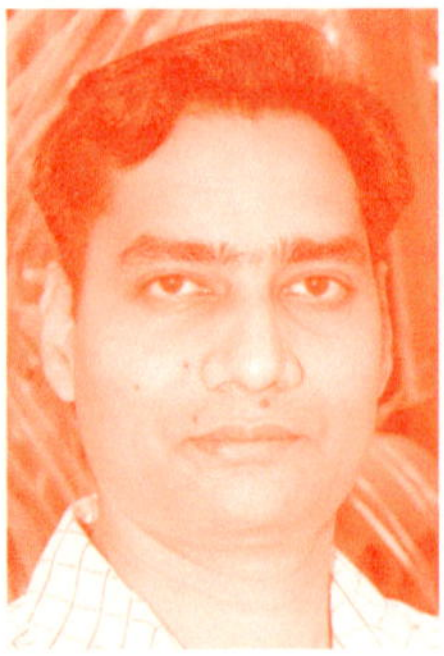
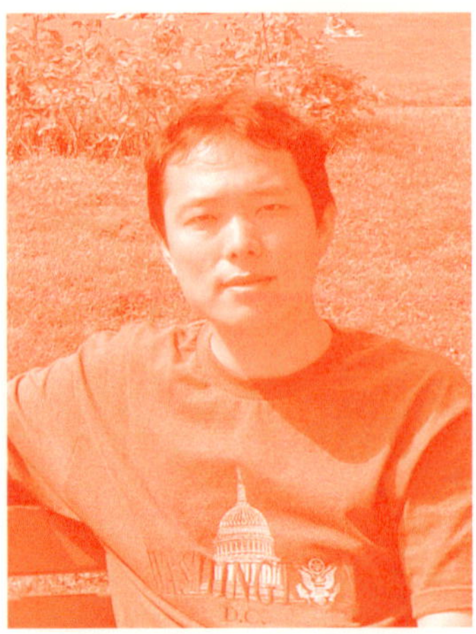
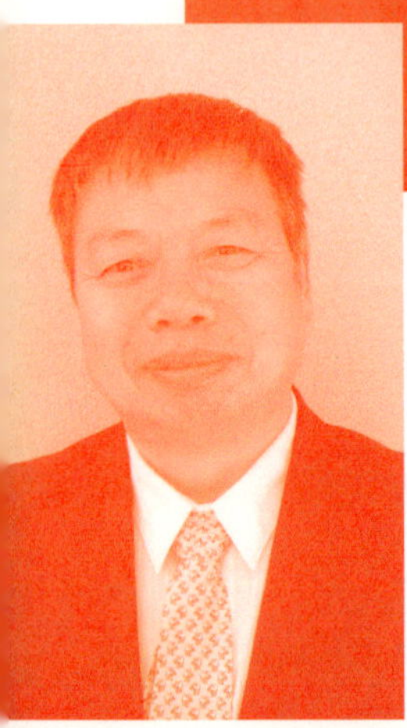
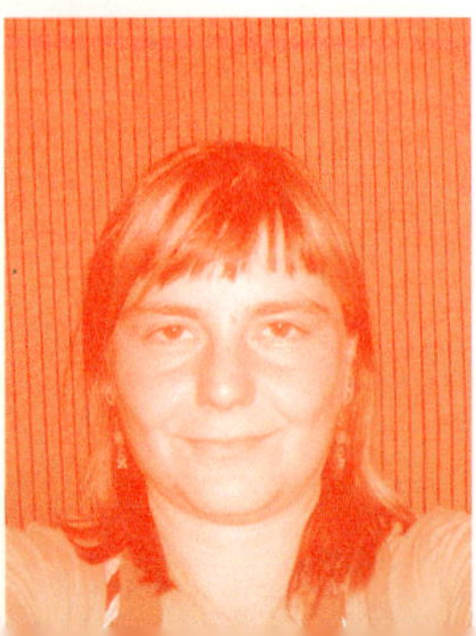

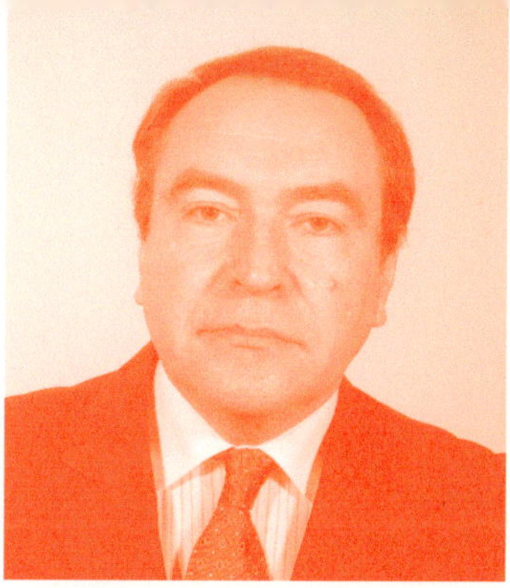
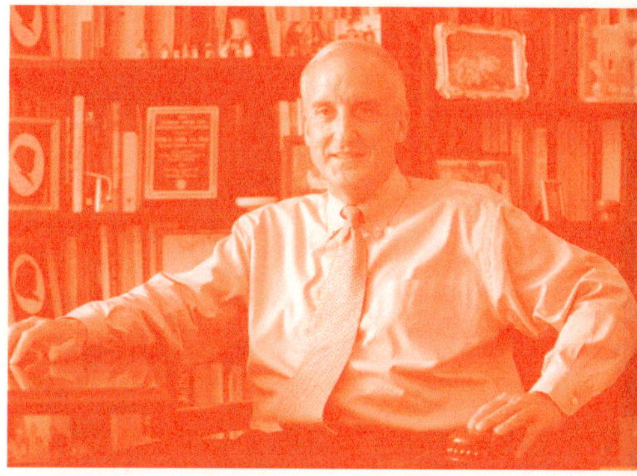
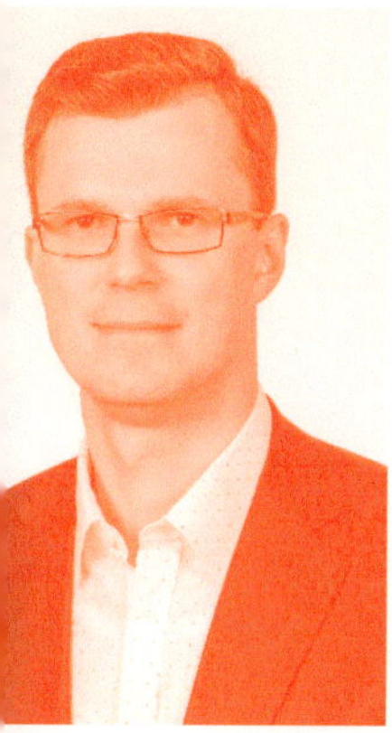
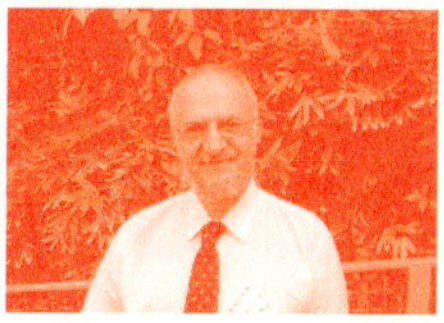
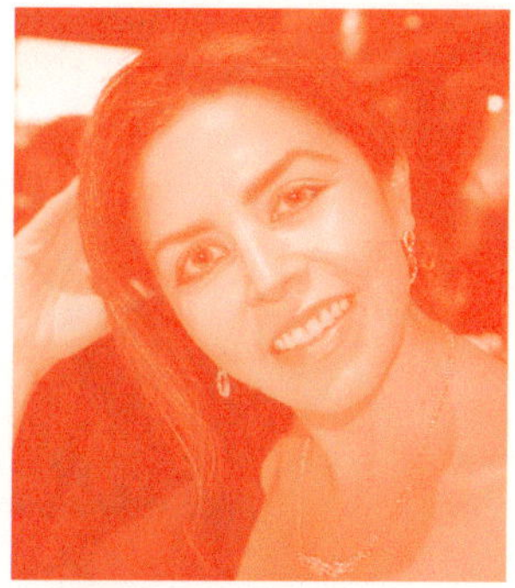

Supporting open minds since 2005

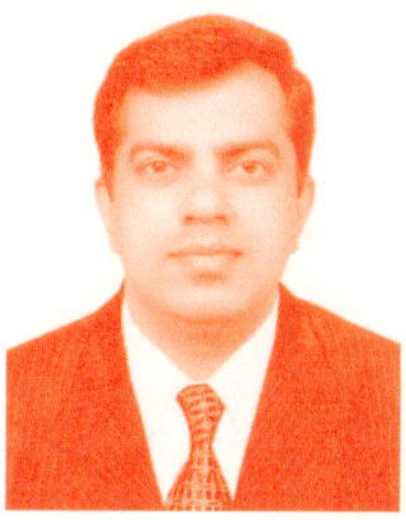
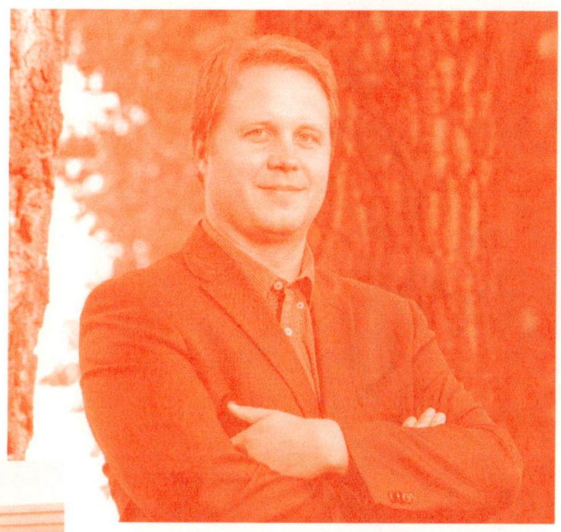
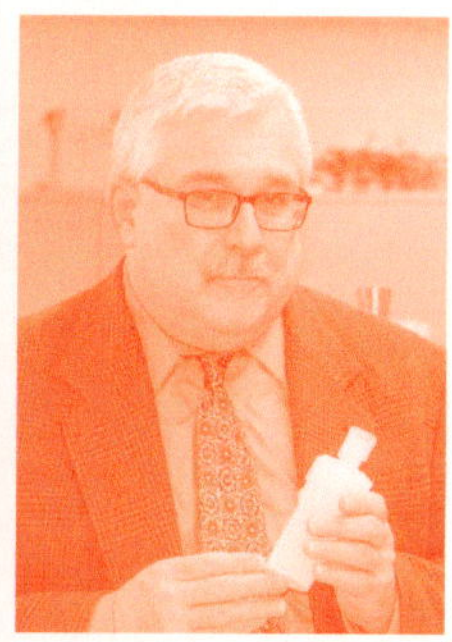
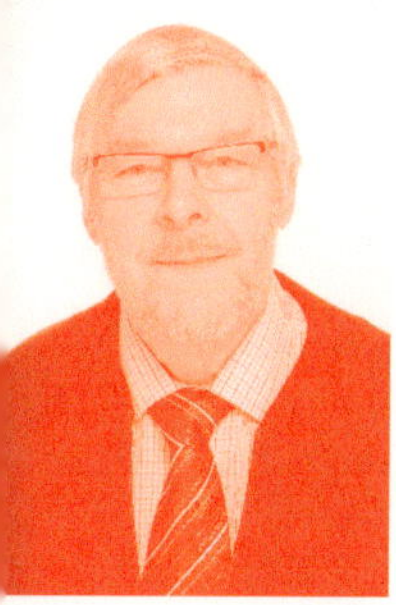
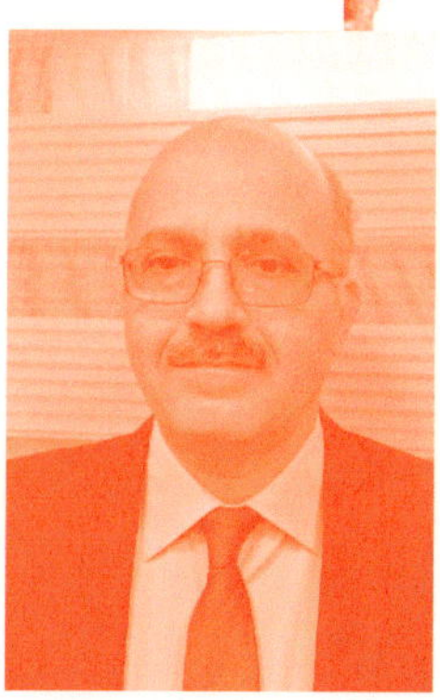
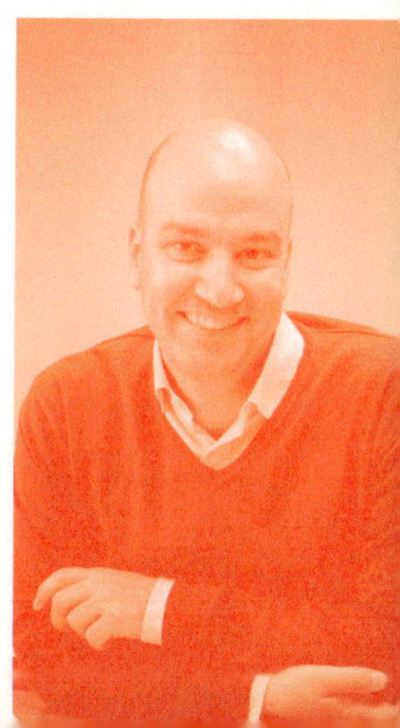
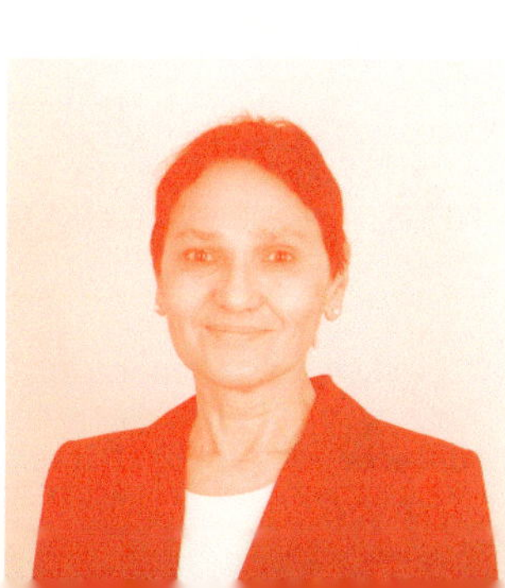

The Current Perspectives on Coronary Artery Bypass Grafting
http://dx.doi.org/10.5772/intechopen.83055
Edited by Takashi Murashita

Contributors
Kiyomi Niki, Motoaki Sugawara, Ahmad Amouzeshi, Zahra Amouzeshi, Maurilio Onofre Deininger, Orlando Oliveira, Daniel Magalhaes, Eugenia Deininger, Mohd. Shahbaaz Khan, Juan Mieres, Hassane Abdallah, Ruchika Meel, S.A. Roohi, Ivana Sopek Merkaš, Nenad Lakušić, Krunoslav Fučkar, Duško Cerovec, Kristina Marić Bešić, Alfredo E. Rodríguez, Ahmed Ibrahim, Khalid Al Khamees

Notice
Statements and opinions expressed in the chapters are these of the individual contributors and not necessarily those of the editors or publisher. No responsibility is accepted for the accuracy of information contained in the published chapters. The publisher assumes no responsibility for any damage or injury to persons or property arising out of the use of any materials, instructions, methods or ideas contained in the book.

First published in London, United Kingdom, 2020 by IntechOpen
IntechOpen is the global imprint of INTECHOPEN LIMITED, registered in England and Wales, registration number: 11086078, 7th floor, 10 Lower Thames Street, London, EC3R 6AF, United Kingdom
Printed in Croatia

British Library Cataloguing-in-Publication Data
A catalogue record for this book is available from the British Library

Additional hard and PDF copies can be obtained from orders@intechopen.com

The Current Perspectives on Coronary Artery Bypass Grafting
Edited by Takashi Murashita
p. cm.
Print ISBN 978-1-78985-965-2
Online ISBN 978-1-78985-966-9
eBook (PDF) ISBN 978-1-83962-857-3

For EU product safety concerns:
IN TECH d.o.o., Prolaz Marije Krucifikse Kozulić 3, 51000 Rijeka, Croatia, info@intechopen.com or visit our website at intechopen.com.

Meet the editor

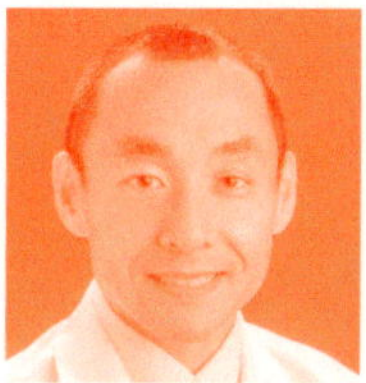

Takashi Murashita, MD, is an assistant professor in the Department of Surgery at the University of Missouri, Columbia, MO, USA. Dr. Murashita received his MD from Kyoto University Medical School, Japan. His main interest is cardiac surgery, and he is a member of the Society of Thoracic Surgery, Eastern Cardiothoracic Surgical Society, and Asian Society for Cardiovascular and Thoracic Surgery. He has published 52 papers in peer-reviewed journals, and 10 book chapters in open access journals. He has been a member of editorial boards for 2 medical journals, and a member of ad-hoc manuscript reviewers for 16 medical journals.

Contents

Preface

This book, "The Current Perspectives on Coronary Artery Bypass Grafting", is an excellent update for health care professionals taking care of patients suffering from severe coronary artery disease. The nine chapters in this book were written by experts in their fields.

The first section describes the hemodynamic mechanism and medical management of coronary artery disease. Chapter 1 discusses the most recent evidence in treating multivessel coronary artery disease and left main coronary artery disease. The author provided a good discussion on the pros and cons of percutaneous coronary intervention versus coronary artery bypass grafting. Chapter 2 and Chapter 4 describe the arterial stiffness and medical therapy in mitral regurgitation associated with coronary artery disease. Chapter 3 gives us a review of antiplatelet therapy after coronary artery bypass grafting. The role of double antiplatelet therapy for percutaneous coronary interventions is well established, whereas its role after surgery remains controversial.

The second section describes technical aspects of coronary artery bypass grafting. Chapter 5 and Chapter 9 describe the technical tips and tricks in surgical anastomosis. These chapters show us a variety of surgical techniques in anastomosing small vessels. Cardiac surgeons should be familiar with multiple anastomotic techniques. Chapter 6 discusses the risk factors that affect early and late survival after coronary artery bypass grafting. Chapter 7 and Chapter 8 discuss the utilization of right internal mammary graft in coronary artery bypass grafting. The benefit of left internal mammary artery graft is well established, whereas the benefit of right internal mammary artery graft remains controversial because of possible increase of sternal infection.

In conclusion, I believe this book will provide health care professionals with the most updated information in the field of surgical intervention for severe coronary artery disease.

Takashi Murashita, MD
Assistant Professor,
Division of Cardiothoracic Surgery,
University of Missouri,
Columbia, MO, USA

Section 1

Mechanism and Management of Coronary Artery Disease

Chapter 1

Current Status, Perspectives, and Future Directions of Multivessel Disease and Left Main Coronary Disease: Its Treatment by PCI or Surgery

Juan Mieres and Alfredo E. Rodríguez

Abstract

MVD has evolved from an era where it was mandatory to treat all lesions, even very thin vessels. With the advent of more realistic anatomical scores such as the ERACI score and the gradient measurements with the fractional flow of reserve (FFR) and instantaneous wave-free ratio (iwFR), a more conservative era has begun, which benefits the patient in the long-term follow-up. The treatment of the LMCA remains a challenging lesion because of the amount of irrigation. It can be divided the treatment of the LMCA with a low or high ERACI score, in the first group is where the PCI has gained in confidence and dedication in addition to knowledge and bifurcation techniques. The second group with high score can only be performed in centers with high PCI experience, since their alternative will always be surgical as the first choice. The revascularization in MVD with STEMI, the priority is the culprit vessel and then evaluate the underlying lesions, an invasive or with a functional test in the short term. The patient with DM is a singular patient, and its treatment should always be evaluated by a multidisciplinary team. We believe that patients with low ERACI score have the possibility of being treated with PCI, but patients with high score are surgical.

Keywords: MVD, PCI, CABG, DM, MI, LMCA, MACCE, BMS, DES

1. Multivessel disease

1.1 Introduction

The revascularization of multivessel disease (MVD) has advanced considerably and has gone through periods where angioplasty with the advent of conventional stents (BMS) was competitive with surgery [1]. After the incorporation of drug-eluting stents (DES) with the significant reduction of the revascularization of the treated vessel, it was thought that the percutaneous coronary intervention (PCI) would be superior to coronary artery bypass graph (CABG), with the advent of the SYNTAX trial [2], which also incorporated an anatomical score that revolutionized the way of stratifying the patients. Although this trial used stents that are not currently marketed, called first-generation DES, later came trials with second-generation stents that also failed to achieve the desired results [3]. An important element was the incorporation of the in vivo functional study of the lesion and its relation with the prognosis, which is the fractional flow of reserve (FFR) [4] and their instantaneous wave-free ratio (iwFR) [5], which gave a physiological view of the coronary disease and its treatment, although its use in stable patients such as the ORBITA trial [6] failed both by design and by results, since 85% of patients are finally revascularized, and the first randomized trial to assess functional lesion testing before CABG found patients who underwent FFR before CABG experienced similar rates of graft failure at 6 months as those who received angiography-guided by surgery [7]. We re-evaluated the SYNTAX score [8] first, and thus we generated an ERACI score [9] more in line with the modern treatment of severe and rational injuries at the time of complete revascularization, targeting medium-to-large caliber vessels, since only 70% lesions were included and vessel lesions larger than 2 mm were included.

1.2 Main trails of PCI vs. CABG and meta-analysis in MVD

In our Argentine Randomized Trial of Coronary Angioplasty With Stenting vs. Coronary Bypass Surgery in Patients With Multivessel Disease (ERACI II) 1, where patients were randomized to PCI with BMS vs. CABG after 5 years of follow-up, there were no significant differences in the mortality of all causes, PCI 7.1% vs. CABG 11.5%, $p = 0.182$. In terms of nonfatal MI, the incidence was 6.2% in the CABG group and 2.8% in the PCI group ($p = 0.128$), where a significant difference was observed in the need for new revascularization, 7.2% in the CABG group and 28.4% in the PCI group ($p = 0.0002$). MACCE was also larger in the PCI group than in the CABG, 24.5% vs. 34.7% ($p = 0.019$). A high rate of patients was asymptomatic without significant differences in both groups. The first randomized trial of patients with first-generation DES vs. CABG and with the creation of an anatomical score to assess severity divided the patients into three groups. This score was based on obstructions of at least 50% in vessels greater than 1.5 mm. Although this very basic score served to stratify patients, the SYNTAX study [2] compared CABG and PCI, followed by placement of paclitaxel-eluting stent in patients with MVD or left main disease (LMCA) or both. At 5 years of follow-up, it was observed that the MACCE between the two groups was significantly higher for the PCI group 37.3% than with the 26.9% CABG ($p < 0.0001$). The MI and the TVR was significantly higher in the PCI group than with surgery, but the mortality of all causes as well as the stroke was not significantly different between the two groups. When analyzed by groups, in the SYNTAX of low score ≤ 22, the MACCE was similar between both groups, but when analyzing intermediate scores 23–32 and high ≥ 33, it was significantly higher with PCI commensurate with CABG. The randomized trial was subsequently carried out with the so-called second-generation DES. In the Randomized CABG and Everolimus-Eluting Stent EES Implantation in the Treatment of Patients with MVD, the BEST trial [3] was performed in 27 sites in East Asia and showed PCI with placement of EES. This study had as its primary end point the composite events of death, MI, and TVR. At 2 years of follow-up, it was observed that there were no significant differences with 11% events in the PCI group compared with 7.9% in the CABG group ($p = 0.32$ for non-inferiority). In the long-term follow-up (4.6 years on average), the events of the primary end point occurred in 15.3% of patients in the PCI group and in 10.6% of those in the CABG group ($p = 0.04$). This is due to an excess of new interventions in the PCI group, since the TVR was significantly higher in the PCI group (11.0% vs. 5.4%, $p = 0.003$). There were no significant differences in mortality between the two groups, 6.6% in the PCI group and

5% in the CABG group (p = 0.30), as well as with the stroke (2.5 and 2.9%, respectively; p = 0.72). The MI was higher in the PCI group than the CABG 4.3% vs. 1.6%, respectively p = 0.02. A recent meta-analysis of Brazilian origin [10] that includes randomized clinical trials (RCT) of multivessel disease performed a group analysis. They identified a total of 15 RCT that satisfied the requirements. The following results were obtained in the pooled data (n = 12,781). Thirty-day mortality and stroke were lower with PCI (1% vs. 1.7%, p = 0.01; and 0.6% vs. 1.7%, p < 0.0001). There was no difference in 1- and 2-year mortality (3.3% vs. 3.7%, p = 0.25; 6.3% vs. 6.0%, p = 0.5). Long-term mortality favored CABG (10.6% vs. 9.4%, p = 0.04), particularly in trials of DES era (10.1% vs. 8.5%, p = 0.01). In diabetics (DM) (n = 3274) long-term mortality favored CABG (13.7% vs. 10.3%, p < 0.0001). In six trials of LMCA (n = 4700), there was no difference in 30-day mortality (0.6% vs. 1.1%, p = 0.15), 1-year mortality (3% vs. 3.7%, p = 0.18), and long-term mortality (8.1% vs. 8.1%) between PCI and CABG. The incidence of stroke was lower with PCI (0.3% vs. 1.5%, p < 0.001). DM and a high SYNTAX score were the subgroups that influenced more adversely the results of PCI (**Table 1**).

1.3 "Functional" complete or anatomic complete revascularization

The fractional flow reserve allows to measure the functional capacity of a stenosis, and if it establishes a threshold of 0.80 (which is equivalent to a maximum intracoronary pressure drop of 20%), it determines a degree of ischemia. In fact, the use of this guide in patients with MVD showed that residual angiographic lesions that were functionally nonsignificant did not cause worse evolution [11] and thus indicated that they do not need treatment, giving a complete revascularization (CR) functional rather than anatomical, since the degree of injury is less important than its functional impact, as well as the magnitude of the territory that irrigates. However, the concept of "functional" CR with PCI was introduced many years ago even when FFR was not available. The ERACI I one of the first randomized clinical trials between PCI and CABG in MVD [12] showed similar outcomes in patients with complete "functional" revascularization achieved with PCI and guided by noninvasive tests and in those with complete "anatomic" revascularization achieved with CABG.

1.4 ERACI risk score

The ERACI IV study [13] was a multicenter, observational, and prospective registry with a second-generation DES in patients with MVD and LMCA. We built a score based on our experience in the treatment of patients with more realistic MVD; since our group led by Dr Rodriguez et al. aimed to treat more critical vessel lesions that irrigate a significant territory, based on this concept we created the ERACI score (ES) by modifying the SYNTAX score (SS), as well as the difference between the treated and residual lesions, their corresponding residual ES or residual SS. This reformulated score included lesions greater than or equal to 70% in vessels larger than 2 mm. The analysis of the bifurcations and CTO was preserved as in the previous score. We included in a novel way the restenosis of the treated vessel that was cataloged as a severely calcified lesion. The rest of the variables were preserved as in the previous score [9] (**Figure 1**). The rationality of this revised score was previously published in our *Journal of Interventional Cardiology* of Argentina (RACI) 3 years ago [9]. With this new modality of scoring with the ES in the ERACI IV study, more than half of the patients had a low ES, and only 17% of the patients had a high score, in contrast to the SS that 34% of the patients were with a high score. The first analysis of this data is that with this score patients are re-categorized into a lower-risk group so they could be treated with either PCI or CABG. When we analyzed the residual untreated

Study	Origin	Date	N	MVD	Characteristics	UA	EF	Off-pump	DM	Outcome
AWESOME [76]	USA	1995–2000	454	2v and 3v	BMS, CABG previous	36	45	0	32	Survival rates for CABG and PCI were 79% versus 80% at 36 months (log-rank test, $p = 0.46$)
ARTS [77, 78]	International	1997–2000	1205	2v and 3v	BMS, majority 2v	30	61	0	21	Event-free survival at 5 years: 58.3% for PCI vs. 78.2% for CABG ($p < 0.0001$)
ERACI II [1]	Argentina	1196–1998	450	2v and 3v	BMS, majority UA	92	ND	0	17	Freedom from MACE at 5 years was lower with PCI than with CABG (65.3% vs. 76.4%; $p = 0.013$)
SOS [79]	Europe and Canada	1995–1999	988	2v and 3v	BMS, majority 2v	33	Nd	3	15	At a median follow-up of 6 years, 53 patients (10.9%) died in the percutaneous coronary intervention group compared with 34 (6.8%) in the CABG group (HR, 1.66; 95% CI, 1.08–2.55; $p = 0.022$)
MASS II [80]	Brazil	1995–2000	408	2v and 3v	BMS, clinical arm	36	65	0	30	The 10-year survival rates were 74.9% with CABG, 75.1% with PCI, and 69% with MT ($p = 0.089$)
LEMANS [29]	Poland	2001–2004	105	LMCAD	BMS and DES, DES if LM < 3.8	32	53	0	25	At 10 years, the mortality of PCI vs. CABG was (21.6% vs. 30.2%; $p = 0.41$) and MACCE (51.1% vs. 64.4%; $p = 0.28$)
SYNTAX [2]	Europe and USA	2005–2007	1800	LM and 3v	DES Taxus	28	Nd	15	35	5-year MACCE in all: 37.3% for PCI vs. 26.9% for CABG ($p < 0.001$) 5-year MACCE in 3 VD: 37.5% for PCI vs. 24.2% for CABG ($p < 0.001$)
CARDia [74]	UK	2002–2007	510	2v and 3v	BMS and DES, only DBT	22	59	31	100	At 1 year of follow-up, the composite rate of death, MI, and stroke was 10.5% in the CABG group and 13.0% in the PCI group (HR, 1.25; 95% CI, 0.75–2.09; $p = 0.39$)
Boudriot et al. [81]	Germany	2003–2009	201	LMCAD	DES (Sirolimus)	ND	ND	46	30	At 1 year of follow-up, the combined primary end point was 13.9% of patients after surgery, as opposed to 19.0% after PCI ($p = 0.19$ for non-inferiority)
PRECOMBAT [28]	Korea	2003–2009	600	LMCAD	DES (Everolimus)	45	60	64	42	At 5 years, MACCE in PCI group and the CABG group (cumulative event rates of 17.5% and 14.3%, respectively; HR, 1.27; 95% CI, 0.84–1.90; $p = 0.26$)

Study	Origin	Date	N	MVD	Characteristics	UA	EF	Off-pump	DM	Outcome
FREEDOM [67]	International	2005–2010	1900	2v and 3v	DES, only DBT	30	65	19	100	The primary outcome occurred more frequently in the PCI group (p = 0.005), with 5-year rates of 26.6% in the PCI group and 18.7% in the CABG group
Va-Cards [73]	USA	2006–2010	198	2v and 3v	DES, only DBT	Nd	Nd	Nd	100	At 2 years, all-cause mortality was 5.0% for CABG and 21% for PCI (HR, 0.30; 95% CI, 0.11–0.80); nonfatal myocardial infarction was 15% for CABG and 6.2% for PCI (HR, 3.32; 95% CI, 1.07–10.30)
BEST [3]	Korea	2008–2013	880	2v and 3v	DES (Everolimus)	42	59	64	45	MACE at 4.6 years: 15.3% for PCI vs. 10.6% for CABG (p = 0.04)
EXCEL [31]	International	2010–2014	1905	LMCAD	DES (Everolimus)	37	57	29	25	At 3 years, a primary end-point event had occurred in 15.4% in the PCI group and in 14.7% in the CABG group (p = 0.02 for non-inferiority; HR, 1.00; 95% CI, 0.79–1.26; p = 0.98 for superiority)
NOBLE [30]	Europe	2008–2015	982	LMCAD	DES (Biolimus)	18	60	16	18	Kaplan-Meier 5-year MACCE was 28% for PCI and 18% for CABG (HR, 1·51; 95% CI, 1·13–2·00; p = 0·0044)

AWESOME, Angina With Extremely Severe Outcomes; ERACI II, Argentine Randomized Study: Coronary Angioplasty With Stenting Versus Coronary Bypass Surgery in Patients With Multivessel Disease; MASS II, Medicine, Angioplasty, or Surgery Study; ARTS, Arterial Revascularization Therapies Study; SOS, Stent or Surgery trial. SYNTAX, Synergy between PCI with Taxus and Cardiac Surgery; CARDia: Coronary Artery Revascularization in Diabetes; Le Mans, Left Main Coronary Artery Stenting; FREEDOM, Future Revascularization Evaluation in Patients with Diabetes Mellitus; Va-Cards, Coronary Artery Revascularization in Diabetes in VA Hospitals; BEST, Bypass Surgery and Everolimus-Eluting Stent Implantation in the Treatment of Patients with Multivessel Coronary Artery Disease; PRECOMBAT, Premier of Randomized Comparison of Bypass Surgery versus Angioplasty Using Sirolimus-Eluting Stent in Patients with Left Main Coronary Artery Disease; EXCEL, Coronary Artery Bypass Surgery for Effectiveness of Left Main Revascularization; NOBLE, Nordic-Baltic-British Left Main Revascularization Study [81]. DES, drug-eluting stents; BMS, bare-metal stent.
Modified from "Stent versus Coronary Artery Bypass Surgery in Multi-Vessel and Left Main Coronary Artery Disease: A Meta-Analysis of Randomized Trials with Subgroups Evaluation" (Pedro José Negreiros de Andrade, João Luiz de Alencar Araripe Falcão, Breno de Alencar Araripe Falcão, Hermano Alexandre Lima Rocha)

Table 1.
Overview of the main trials of MVCAD and LMCAD.

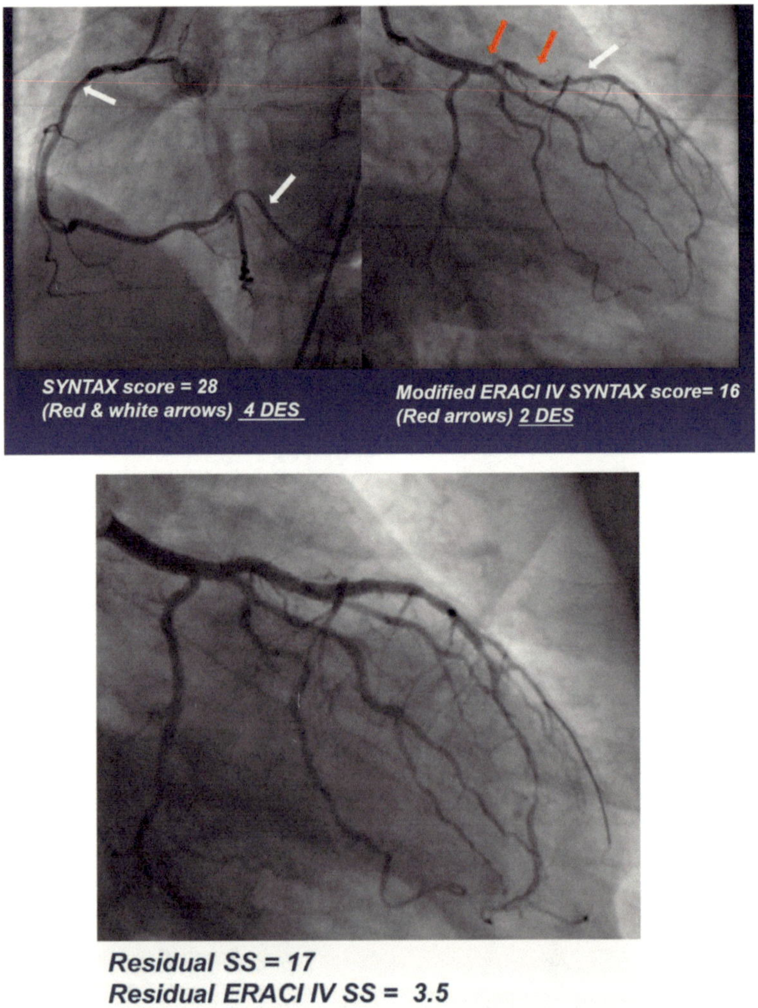

Figure 1.
Modification of the SYNTAX score by ERACI score, with residual SYNTAX and ERACI scores and its implications. SYNTAX score = 28 points (red and white arrows). Hypothetically the patients need 4 DES. Modified ERACI score, in the ERACI IV, the SYNTAX score (only the red arrows) was 16 points = patient received 2 DES. The residual ERACI score was 3.5. If the patient was scored with the SYNTAX score, he would have had 17 residual SYNTAX score.

lesions between these two scores, we also found significant differences between these two groups of patients since with RSS it was 8.7 ± 5.9 vs. and with RES it was 3.5 ± 4.6, $p = 0.003$. In addition, reasonably incomplete revascularization was defined, defined by a residual of ≤5 (**Table 2**). If we take the RSS, only 35% of the patients reached this goal, but if we analyze it with the RES, they reached 80%, which suggests that most patients achieved a functional rather than an anatomical revascularization (**Table 2**). This could be corroborated in the long-term follow-up where these patients had a MACCE less than 10% at 3 years of follow-up. In addition, this score was validated in another trial of our group called the WALTZ registry [14]. A total of 201 real-life patients were included prospectively, in 11 centers in the Argentine Republic using the same criteria of ERACI IV. The study design, as well as the rationale, was previously published [15]. When we performed the analysis regarding the scores, we found a significant difference with respect to the baseline (SS 11.8 + 6.8 vs. ES 7.8 + 5.3, $p = 0.0016$), and the same happened with the residual (RSS 5.4 + 5.6 vs. RES 1.3 + 2.9, $p < 0.001$). The analysis that we carry out is that the presence of

	SYNTAX score	ERACI score	P value
Number of patients (n)	225	225	
Low group	33.8%	54.8%	< 0.001
Intermediate group	32.4%	27.9%	= 0.35
High group	33.8%	17.2%	<0.001
Baseline mean	27.7 ± 11.3	22 ± 11.02	=0.0004
Residual mean	8.7 ± 5.9	3.5 ± 4.6	=0.003
Residual ≤5	35%	80%	<0.001
Residual <8	48%	93.5%	=0.002

From "Lowering Risk Score Profile During PCI in Multiple Disease is Associated with Low Adverse Events: The ERACI Risk Score" (Alfredo E. Rodriguez, Carlos Fernandez-Pereira, Juan Mieres, Hernan Pavlovsky, Juan del Pozo, Alfredo M. Rodriguez-Granillo, David Antoniucci, On behalf of ERACI IV Investigators)

Table 2.
Differences in baseline and residual risk scores: ERACI IV registry.

neoatherosclerosis [16] that we believe is also present in the second- and third-generation stents is a growing concern, which is why this more rational strategy of the use of these devices can lead to better results long term. When we look closely at the results of the Syntax II study where iwFR was used, we can verify that the conservative strategy is beneficial [17]. When we compare the PCI group guided by the iwFR with the SYNTAX I in the PCI group, we find a decrease in MI and MACCE, similar to the SYNTAX I CABG group. SYNTAX II treated fewer lesions per patient than SYNTAX I (2.6 vs. 4, $p < 0.001$) and then implanted fewer stents per patient (3.8% vs. 5.2%, $p < 0.001$) despite the fact that the two groups of patients were scored similarly, with SS ($p = 0.16$). These results are consistent with our ERACI IV trial. We also have to recognize that the FFR analysis has numerous limitations, among them it can be technically difficult in segments of diffuse disease, tandem lesions and bifurcation lesions. When performed in patients with severe aortic stenosis, the evaluation is more complex to analyze. Also you have to assume the cost of catheters that cannot be ignored. It is also important to mention that studies of CABG guided by FFR [18] have not achieved the expected results when compared when guided by angiography, and studies such as FAME 2 comparing optimal medical treatment vs. guided PCI have not observed reduction in MI or long-term mortality [19].

1.5 Guidelines

The evidence suggests that in MVD without DM and low anatomical complexity, PCI and CABG achieve similar long-term outcomes with respect to survival and the composite of death, MI, and stroke, justifying a class I recommendation for PCI. Consistent results were also obtained for patients with MVD in the recent individual patient-level meta-analysis. Thus, the previous class III recommendation for PCI in MVD and intermediate-to-high complexity was maintained [20]. The intermediate and high SYNTAX scores are associated with better evolution with the CABG. Although this score is very limited and impractical for its application, its use for making decisions in patients with MVD is reasonable [21]. The ERACI score could be more rational for making decisions due to being more realistic and conservative [9].

1.6 Ongoing trials

The Prospective Multicenter Registry of Hybrid Coronary Artery Revascularization Combined with Surgical Bypass and Percutaneous Coronary Intervention Using

Everolimus-Eluting Metallic Stents evaluates the efficacy of hybrid coronary revascularization (HCR) combining CABG and PCI in the treatment of MVD. CABG is to be performed in the left anterior descending artery and the left circumflex artery using only arterial grafts, whereas PCI is to be conducted for the treatment of the right coronary artery with everolimus-eluting stents (EESs) [22]. The Comparison of One-stop Hybrid Revascularization vs. Off-pump Coronary Artery Bypass for the Treatment of Multi-vessel Disease combines minimally invasive direct CABG and PCI to be performed in the hybrid operating suite, an enhanced operating room equipped with radiographic capability [23].

1.7 Conclusions

In our long experience in the treatment of MVD for more than two decades and according to our score, we believe that the stratified treatment can be divided into two groups, patients with low and intermediate scores in whom the results of PCI are comparable with surgery. The other group of patients are those with high scores, we think that the current state-of-the-art CABG is the treatment of choice. However, with the increase in stent technology this difference can be reduced.

2. Left main coronary artery disease

2.1 Introduction

LMCA is a disease with significant morbidity and mortality, since it threatens a large myocardial territory. LMCA stenosis occurs in approximately 15% of patients with symptomatic ischemic heart disease [24]. The most common cause of LMCA disease is atherosclerosis, which is rarely focal and involves bifurcation in 80% of cases, which usually extends from the LMCA to the LAD [25]. In the beginning, the treatment of choice for this disease was the CABG [26]. However, after the introduction of PCI, there was a growing interest in the treatment of the LMCA. Both European [20] and American [21] guidelines recommend CABG (class I) as the treatment of choice for LMCA in patients with low risk score. These recommendations were based mainly on the results of the LMCA subgroup analysis of the SYNTAX trial (705 patients) that showed no differences in the MACCE between CABG and PCI in patients with LM disease [27]. Patients treated with PCI had a lower stroke but a higher revascularization rate than CABG. The results of the PRECOMBAT trial [28] compare PCI to CABG in the treatment of LMCA. The two groups did not differ significantly in MACCE. Ischemia-driven revascularization occurred more frequently in the PCI group than in the CABG group. In addition, the LE MANS trial [29] with a 10-year follow-up compared PCI and CABG in patients with LMCA with low or medium SYNTAX score. The primary end point was the left ventricular ejection fraction (LVEF) that was slightly higher in the PCI group than the CABG group. The introduction of new-generation DES with proven efficacy and safety prompted the design of two large randomized trials: the Nordic-Baltic-British Left Main Revascularization Study (NOBEL) [30] and the Evaluation of Xience versus Coronary artery bypass surgery for Effectiveness of Left main revascularization (EXCEL) trial [31]. It is important to note that, when an LMCA PCI is performed, there is a greater awareness of the need to achieve optimal procedural results by using the available technologies, including the most effective stents, intravascular evaluation of image, and physiology. And when one faces a real bifurcation with a Medina classification [32], it is necessary to use two stents. It would seem that the best technique is double kissing balloon with crush (DKC) [33].

2.2 Main trials of the LMCA

LE MAS trial, [29] in this prospective, multicenter trial, randomly assigned 105 patients with LMCA with low and medium complexity of coexisting coronary artery disease according to SYNTAX score to PCI with stenting (n = 52) or CABG (n = 53). DES were implanted in 35%, whereas arterial grafts to the left anterior descending artery were utilized in 81%. This study is very interesting because it offers a 10-year follow-up, which as a primary end point was the evaluation of the ejection fraction between PCI and CABG in the treatment of LMCA. Although there were no significant differences, there was a tendency in favor of PCI (54.9 ± 8.3% vs. 49.8 ± 10.3%, p = 0.07). Regarding mortality, MI, and TVR, there were no statistical differences between the two groups, although there was also a trend of greater MACCE-free survival in the PCI group (34.7% vs. 22.1%, p = 0.06; reason risk, 1.71; 95% confidence interval (CI), 0.97–2.99). The Nordic-Baltic-British Left Main Revascularization Study [30] is a prospective, randomized, open-label, non-inferiority trial done at 36 centers in Europe. Patients were randomized to CABG or PCI. LMCA were visually assessed with diameter ≥ 50% or fractional flow reserve ≤0.80 in different segments of the left main coronary artery. SYNTAX score was calculated and all patients with low, medium, and high score were included. Patients were treated with the intention of achieving CR. Biolimus-eluting stent was the recommended stent in this trial. Distal bifurcation lesions could be treated with various techniques preferably by the "culotte" technique. IVUS was strongly recommended pre- and post-stent deployment. In the CABG group, the left internal mammary artery was recommended for revascularization of the left anterior descending coronary artery, and for the other lesions, saphenous venous grafts, free arterial grafts, or the right internal mammary artery could be used. The primary end point was a MACCE. About 1184 patients were included in the analysis (592 patients in each group). The SYNTAX scores were similar between the two groups (22.4 in the PCI group and 22.3 in the CABG group). CABG was performed with the on-pump technique in 84% of patients, and 96% of patients underwent arterial grafting of the left anterior descending artery. Kaplan-Meier estimates of MACCE were significantly higher in PCI (28%) than in CABG (18%). The rate of MI and revascularization was significantly higher in PCI group than in CABG, but the overall mortality and stroke were not statistically significant. At 30 days, the stroke rate in PCI group was significantly less than in the CABG group, but this difference was not seen at 1- and 5-year follow-up. The EXCEL trial [31] was a prospective randomized open-label, non-inferiority trial undertaken at 126 centers in 17 countries around the world. Patients were randomized to receive either CABG or PCI. Patients who had stable and unstable angina were included in the study; however patient who were having MI were excluded. Patients were included if they had LMCA of 70% assessed visually or 50–70% determined by means of invasive or noninvasive methods. SYNTAX score was determined and patients who had score of higher than 33 were excluded. CR was the intention of treatment in both groups. A second-generation DES EES was used in this study. Distal bifurcating lesions were treated with a two-stent strategy using various techniques. CABG was performed both on- and off-pump, with the aim of CR for vessels with 50% stenosis. Arterial grafts were strongly recommended. The primary end point was MACCE at 3 years. The intention-to-treat (ITT) analysis was used in this trial. A total of 1905 patients underwent randomization, 948 were assigned to the PCI group and 957 to the CABG group. The SYNTAX score according to assessment at local sites was low (≤22) in 60.5% of the patients and intermediate (23–32) in 39.5% of the patients. Distal LMCA was present in 80.5% of the patients. IVUS imaging guidance was used in nearly 80% of the patients in the PCI group. There was no difference between the two groups in respect to the primary composite end-point event of death, stroke, or myocardial infarction at 3 years (15.4% of the patients in the PCI group and in 14.7% of the patients in the CABG group). At 3 years, the composite end-point event of death, stroke, myocardial infarction, or ischemia-driven revascularization had occurred in 23.1% of the patients in the PCI group and in 19.1% of the patients in the CABG group. Ischemia-driven revascularization during follow-up was more frequent after PCI than after CABG (in 12.6% vs. 7.5% of the patients, $p < 0.001$). Stent thrombosis occurred in only 0.7% of patients within 3 years after the procedure and was less common than symptomatic graft occlusion. In the Premier of Randomized comparison of Bypass surgery versus Angioplasty using Sirolimus-Eluting Stent in Patients with Left Main Coronary Artery Disease (PRECOMBAT) [28] trial was a randomized study where 600 patients with LMCA went to PCI with a first-generation of DES or CABG. The primary end point was the combined events, MACCE, at 5 years of follow-up 17.5% were observed in the PCI and 14.3 % in the CABG group, $p = 0.26$. Regarding the mortality of all causes, MI or stroke, there were no significant differences. The TVR was more frequent with PCI than with CABG (11.4% vs. 5.5%, $p = 0.012$).

2.3 Analysis of the two principal trials

As we could see in these last two studies on PCI and CABG in the LMCA, we can see that the NOBLE [30] study included higher-risk patients and used a pharmacological stent with biodegradable polymer. In addition to the fact that the most frequently used technique was "culotte" by recommendation, the use of IVUS was only 75% in post PCI patients, and only 55% of the kissing balloon was performed. In addition the use of the proximal optimization (POT) was not specified, and first-generation stent was also used in 8% of patients. In the EXCEL study [31], a second-generation stent was used in patients with low and intermediate SYNTAX scores, and the amount of IVUS used reached 77%. The use of POT was also not specified, no special bifurcation technique was recommended, and the use of kissing balloon was also not specified (**Table 3**).

2.4 Meta-analysis

The objective was to compare clinical results and safety during short- and long-term follow-up by conducting a meta-analysis of large pooled data from randomized controlled trials and updated observation. The primary outcome was MACCE, MI, stroke, all-cause mortality, and revascularization after at least 1 year of follow-up. A subgroup analysis was also performed with a follow-up of over 5 years. A total of 29 studies with 21,832 patients (10,424 with PCI and 11,408 with CABG) were analyzed. At 1-year follow-up there was a significant difference in favor of the CABG in MACCE, TVR, and MI, but the stroke was significantly lower in the PCI group. In the 5-year group analysis, it showed similar results except that the MACCE showed no inferiority in the PCI group. This meta-analysis concludes that the PCI for the LMCA can be applied in carefully selected patients. The MI and the TVR remain worrying, although we must consider that most of these studies have used first-generation DES [34].

2.5 PCI strategy and technique

Angioplasty is a specialty where the practice generates a greater capacity to solve problems during the procedure. It has been seen that those operators who perform at least 15 PCI of LMCA per year in 3 consecutive years obtain better results [35].

	EXCEL	NOBLE
Inclusion criteria	- Unprotected left main coronary artery (ULMCA) disease or left main equivalent disease - Clinical and anatomic eligibility for both PCI and CABG as agreed to by the local heart team - Silent ischemia, stable angina, unstable angina, recent MI with normalization of CK-MB prior randomization - In addition to randomized patients, it also includes universal registry	- Stable, unstable angina pectoris, or acute coronary syndrome - Significant ULMCA with no more than three additional noncomplex PCI lesions - Patient eligible to be treated by CABG and by PCI
Main exclusion criteria	- Prior PCI of the left main at any time prior to randomization or prior PCI of any other (non-left main) coronary artery lesions within 1 year prior to randomization - Prior CABG - Need for any concomitant cardiac surgery - Inability to receive dual antiplatelet therapy for at least 1 year - Pregnancy or intention to become pregnant - Life expectancy less than 3 years	- ST elevation infarction within 24 h - Patient is too high risk for CABG - Expected survival less than 1 year - Allergy to aspirin, clopidogrel, or ticlopidine
Angiographic exclusion criteria	SYNTAX score ≥ 33 - Visually estimated left main reference vessel diameter < 2.25 mm or > 4.25 mm (post-dilatation up to 4.5 mm is allowed)	- CABG clearly better treatment option (LMCA stenosis and > 3 or complex additional coronary lesions)
Primary end point	- Death, MI, and stroke	- Death, stroke, non-procedural MI, and new revascularization (PCI or CABG)
Sample size	1.905	1200
Participating centers	131	36
Main results	At 3 years, a primary end-point event had occurred in 15.4% of the patients in the PCI group and in 14.7% of the patients in the CABG group	At 5 years, primary end points occurred in 28% of the patients in PCI group and in 18% of the patients in the CABG group
Conclusion	In patients with left main coronary artery disease and low or intermediate SYNTAX scores, PCI was non-inferior to CABG	CABG might be better than PCI for treatment of left main stem coronary artery disease

Modified from "NOBLE and EXCEL: The debate for excellence in dealing with left main stenosis" (Hamood Al Kindi, Amir Samaan, Hatem Hosny)

Table 3.
Comparison of EXCEL and NOBLE trials.

The PCI of the ostium and the middle third of the LMCA is technically easier if we analyze it by the ERACI score this doesn't give more than 5 points, unlike the distal third that compromises ostium of the two coronaries and presents higher ERACI scores [36]. When one faces the distal third of the LMCA, there is a totally different approach. Anyway there are different types of bifurcations, where we prefer to use the Medina classification [32]. To assess them, the provisional stent technique has become a technique with a lot of boom and has had good results compared to techniques with two stents [37]. The technique of the provisional stent has been used in up to two thirds of the branches of the LMCA. However, after two RCTs where the DKC was used as a technique, these tests presented better results than the culotte technique or the provisional stent for the treatment of bifurcations with Medina 1,1,1 or 0,1,1 [33, 38]. In both studies, a reduction in ischemic events was observed. The decision to use a bifurcation technique with one or two stents is basically in the exact evaluation of the compromise of the origin of the left coronary circumflex or the left coronary ramus in a trifurcation. The best way to assess these vessels is with the images of the IVUS or the optimal coherence tomography (OCT) [39]. When the provisional stent technique is used and a residual obstruction of around 50% is observed, the measurement with functional study with iwFR or FFR could be considered as a complement in the decision-making of its definitive treatment. The use of kissing balloon and POT has been invoked as optimizers for this complex carrefour. Also, the post-stent images or stents of both the IVUS and the OCT are important when making decisions, since these elements clearly inform two elements that are key such as uncovered dissections or stent not well positioned [40]. The technique used in the treatment of LMCA is extremely important, just as training in true bifurcation is also difficult. Patients with true bifurcation are those who have Medina 1,1,1 or 0,1,1 and should be treated with two stents and we believe that the technique of choice is DKC. Another important element is to only include patients with low and intermediate ERACI score [17] and leave patients with high scores for very selected centers and true contraindication or patients who really refuses surgery. The use of images in diagnosis, implantation, and postimplantation has become a mandatory strategy, including the use of IVUS and optimal coherence tomography [41]. An element that has been incorporated into the technical arsenal is the technique of proximal optimization. The proximal optimization technique is a key part of treating large bifurcation lesions and will optimize results of both single- and two-stent strategies. An appropriately sized balloon should be positioned and inflated just up to the carina. When performed well, the enhanced lesion scaffolding, reduced strut mal-apposition, and improved flow dynamics are likely to translate into improved clinical results [42].

2.6 Guidelines

The evidence is clear regarding patients with low scores, where treatment with both PCI and CABG is appropriate, where there is a class I recommendation. In patients with high scores, because the evidence is much lower because many of these patients have been excluded from RCTs, the recommendation for PCI is class III, since the benefit is clearly greater with CABG. In patients with intermediate scores, due to the lack of evidence in the long-term follow-up, the recommendation remains IIa [20, 43]. When one makes a global evaluation of the LMCA and addresses the guidelines, one must also take into consideration the different portions of the LMCA such as the ostium, the middle third, and the distal third, since they have different implications, both in the technique and in the evolution of these patients, so they would probably have to be analyzed separately. Also the degree of angiographic stenosis has been changing and should not be left with the 50% obstruction that has been used universally, and perhaps it should be passed at least 70%. Although this analysis can have many deficiencies, the use of images such as IVUS or OCT or even functional studies with iwFR or FFR can be closer to a true significant obstruction. It is believed that a minimum luminal diameter of 2.8 mm or an area of $< 6\ mm^2$ would suggest a physiologically significant obstruction [21].

2.7 Ongoing trials

Xience versus Synergy in LMCA PCI (ideal-LM), PCI of the LMCA a comparison of the newest generation of DES in combination with a short duration of

DAPT. The additional use of OCT image can be considered a standard procedure with a very low risk of major complications 0.4% [44]. VeRy thin Stents for Patients with Left mAIN or bifurcation in real life: the RAIN Multicenter Study, for coronary stents, reducing the thickness of the struts has become one of the most important innovations, since it is related to easier crushability and reduced risk of thrombosis and low rate of TVR. They performed a multicenter registry of patients treated with Biomatrix flex, Xience Alpine, Ultimaster, Resolute Onyx and Synergy. MACCE (death, MI, TLR and stent thrombosis) will be the primary end point [45].

2.8 Conclusions

In the treatment of severe LMCA in patients with low to intermediate ERACI score, the percutaneous treatment is of choice. In those with a higher score or who have total occlusions and are DM, surgical treatment is better. It is very important to evaluate each case in particular as well as work with a heart team to discuss cases that may generate controversy. The interventional cardiology must be trained in the different bifurcation techniques as well as have images such as IVUS or OCT for procedures. The implementation of the final kissing balloon and the POT in all patients is important. DKC seems to be the technique of choice in LMCA diseases with true bifurcations.

3. Patients with STEMI and MVD

3.1 Introduction

About half of the patients who enter with acute myocardial infarction with ST segment elevation (STEMI) have MVD [46]. Although it seems logical that patients with MVD have a worse prognosis, due to the extent of coronary lesions manifested by higher scores, this remains controversial. There are elements that determine that lesions at multiple sites of the coronary arteries can be complicated, and there are studies in which the multivessel PCI shows a better evolution compared to patients in whom they only receive treatment of the culprit vessel, although there are other studies they don't confirm it and consider them innocent [47], and therefore these arteries warrant treatment in much the same way one would approach any unstable lesion. An update on primary PCI for patients with STEMI (class IIb) [20, 48] by the guidelines recommends intervention of the non-culprit at the time of primary PCI if the patient is hemodynamically stable before the discharge. Subsequently, two randomized trials showed that treatment of non-culprit lesions in the acute phase reduced the risk of future adverse events. The PRAMI trial [49], CvlPRIT trial [50], and recently DANAMI-3-PRIMULTI trial [51] studied the clinical outcomes by comparing the FFR guided by CR with culprit-only PCI in STEMI and found that the composite rate of all-cause mortality, nonfatal reinfarction, and repeat revascularization was significantly lower in the CR group, which was mainly driven by a reduction in repeat revascularization. More recently, another randomized trial (COMPARE ACUTE) [52] revealed that FFR-guided complete revascularization of non-culprit arteries in an acute setting was associated with a lower risk of the composite cardiovascular outcome. We emphasized the importance of individualizing care for each patient, balancing the anticipated benefits from multivessel PCI against the potential risks.

3.2 Complete vs. incomplete revascularization

Data derived from more than 150,000 patients undergoing PCI suggest that less than 50% of all patients with MVD have CR after they have undergone percutaneous revascularization. It was observed that CR is associated with a fall in the incidence of mortality, MI, and MACCE, regardless of whether an anatomical or functional definition was used for the evaluation of IR, and perhaps the degree CR is associated with the magnitude of the risk. The association between IR and adverse clinical outcomes suggests that in patients with MVD, the degree of CR that can be achieved by PCI should be considered when discussing the choice of revascularization modality with the heart team, in addition to considering the complexity of the injury, functional significance, patient characteristics, and ERACI score [9, 53].

3.3 Randomized trials

The preventive angioplasty in acute myocardial infarction (PRAMI) study [49] was performed in five centers in the United Kingdom in patients with STEMI and MVD, where they were randomized to preventive angioplasty of non-culprit vessels vs. only PCI of the culprit vessel. It was the first of the trials that incorporated a new concept on complete revascularization in STEMI and MVD. At practically 2 years of follow-up, a reduction of more than 50% was observed on the primary end point that was the combined event of cardiac death, nonfatal MI, and refractory angina, of the patients of the preventive PCI group vs. PCI only of the culprit vessel. The study was designed to include 600 patients but was stopped early with 465 patients because the data was conclusive by the data security committee. CvLPRIT [50] (trial of primary PCI vs. complete primary injury) compared a multivessel PCI strategy in patients with STEMI (performed at the time of primary PCI or revascularization in stages before discharge) to revascularization of culprit-vessel only. In this trial, 7 centers in the United Kingdom participated, where 296 patients were included, randomization was performed by stratification between previous or non-previous infarction, and according to the time ≤3 or >3 h. The primary end point of the study was the combined events of all-cause mortality, recurrent MI, heart failure, or revascularization driven by 12-month ischemia. The result produced a reduction of primary events to more than half in the CR group (10 vs. 21%; hazard ratio (HR), 0.45; 95% CI, 0.24–0.84; $p = 0.009$). There were no differences in individual events. In the compare acute study [52] (multivessel angioplasty guided by fractional flow reserve in myocardial infarction), they included 885 patients in 24 centers in Asia and Europe, where patients with STEMI and MVD, after a primary PCI stable, were randomized to complete revascularization guided by FFR of the artery not culprit of all lesions greater than 50% vs. angioplasty only of the culprit vessel. The FFR was performed in both groups, but its results were blind to operators and patients in the culprit vessel group only. The primary end point of the study was the MACCE at 1 year, which was significantly better in the FFR-guided group (7.8% vs. 20.5%) than in the culprit vessel only (HR, 0.35; 95% CI, 0.22–0.55; $p < 0.001$). This was at the expense of revascularization without changes in mortality or MI. The DANAMI-3-PRIMULTI [51] (The Third Danish Study of Optimal Acute Treatment of Patients With STEMI: Primary PCI in Multivessel Disease) was conducted at two university centers in Denmark, where they randomized 627 patients with STEMI and MVD after a successful primary PCI of the culprit vessel to a complete revascularization guided by FFR compared to conservative treatment. The primary end point was MACCE, which was composed of death, nonfatal MI, and revascularization driven by ischemia. After an average follow-up of 27 months, it was observed that the FFR group presented a MACCE of 13% vs. 22% in conservative treatment (HR, 0.56; 95%

CI, 0.38–0.83; p = 0.004). This result was due to an excess of revascularization driven by ischemia in the conservative group. In the PRAGUE-13 trial [54], Ota Hlinomaz et al. in a university hospital in the Czech Republic randomized 214 patients with STEMI and MVD, who had an obstruction of at least ≥70%, to a group with CR day 3–40 after primary PCI compared with conservative treatment, where the primary end point was MACCE that was composed of death from all causes, nonfatal MI, and stroke, and after a mean of 38 months showed no significant differences in both groups, (16% in CR vs. 13.9 in conservative treatment; HR, 1.35; 95% CI, 0.66–2.74; p = 0.407). CULPRIT-SHOCK [55] was a study that surprised in terms of results and gave new directives in the treatment that we had been doing in this pathology, this multicenter study was carried out in 83 centers in Europe that included 706 patients with cardiogenic shock, with SETEMI and NSTEMI, at CR compared to the treatment of the culprit vessel only (CVO), whose primary end point was mortality and renal failure with dialysis at 30 days. The combined event occurred in 55.4 in the CR vs. 45.9% in the treatment of the CVO, (relative risk, 0.83; 95% CI, 0.71–0.96; p = 0.01). A significant difference in mortality between the two groups was also observed (CR 51.5 vs. CVO 43.3%; relative risk, 0.84; 95% CI, 0.72–0.98; p = 0.03).

3.4 Score to evaluate the treatment in MVD with MI

Hae Chang Jeong et al., developed a new Score to predict combined events in patients with AMI and MVD, the CONVERSE score, based on the PCI registry of nine centers in universities in Korea, in a registry of 5025 patients, evaluated 2630 patients who AMI and MVD had presented, and they were divided into two groups those who were treated CVO that were 1029 patients vs. those with PCI of MVD 1601, for this they used 8 variables that had been predictors of events in a previous study [56]. The variables were patients with arterial hypertension, diabetes, age over 65 years, deterioration of EF, heart failure in presentation, chronic renal failure, elevated CRP plasmatic, anterior descending or LMCA as culprit vessel, each variable awarded a point, the elevation above 3 points in these patients were in linear relationship with the elevation of the MACCE [57].

3.5 Meta-analysis of MVD in STEMI

In this meta-analysis of 10 trials with 2285 patients. Among the three complete revascularization strategies, that is, during the procedure index, during hospitalization or after discharge vs. treatment of the culprit vessel only, it was associated with MACCE reduction (reference rate ratio [RR], 0.57; 95% CI, 0.42–0.77), due to a lower rate of emergency revascularization. Mortality of all causes and spontaneous reinfarction was similar between the two groups. There were no differences between the different types of strategies at the time of revascularization in patients with CR [58].

3.6 An algorithm for the management of STEMI patients with MVD

Figure 2 [59].

3.7 Guidelines

MVD PCI treatment during STEMI is considered strongly indicated when there are critical lesions or associated thrombotic lesions when the culprit vessel has already been treated if there is persistent ischemia. When there is cardiogenic shock, the only treatment of the culprit vessel is the treatment of choice [20]. Patients with stable STEMI and MVD after a primary PCI the recommendation of multivessel PCI

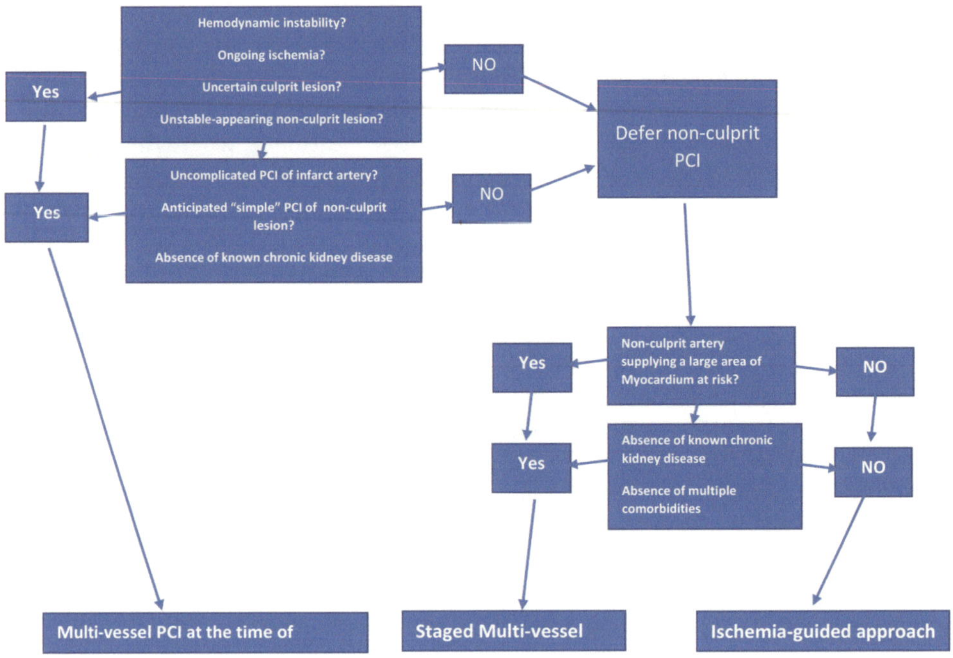

Figure 2.
Algorithm for the Management of STEMI Patients With MVD. Modified from "The Management of MVD in STEMI: The Science and Art of Decision-Making in STEMI" (Feb 07, 2018) (Jacqueline E. Tamis-Holland, MD, FACC; Addi Suleiman, MBBS).

has been updated to a Class IIB, this could be done at the time of the primary index or in stages during hospitalization or after discharge [48].

3.8 Ongoing trials

The COMPLETE [60] (Complete vs. Culprit-only Revascularization to Treat Multi-vessel Disease After Primary PCI for STEMI) trial will compare the outcomes of approximately 3900 patients randomized to a strategy of staged multivessel PCI or culprit-only revascularization. The FULL REVASC [61] (FFR-Guidance for Complete Non-Culprit Revascularization) This trial intends to evaluate the CR in about 4000 patients with STEMI or not with very high risk in patients of MVD guided by FFR during the same hospitalization of the index procedure, to evaluate clinical results.

3.9 Our experience

We were the precursors in the treatment of primary PCI in acute infarction as revealed by one of the first randomized trials with stent in acute myocardial infarction, our trial GRAMI [62]. In our daily practice we try to identify culprit vessel. If we have a territory where we find two vessels with critical lesions, we treat them. If the patient presents a critical lesion in another territory, we defer to perform it pre-discharge. We also consider the amount of territory that this vessel irrigates as well as its renal function when making the decision with the heart team.

3.10 Conclusions

Multivessel PCI both during the index procedure and in stages in stable patients is safe and could lead to better long-term results at the expense of reducing emergency revascularization without altering mortality. The PCI of associated intermediate or very complex lesions at the time of STEMI is contraindicated. In cardiogenic shock and MVD, the treatment of the culprit vessel is only the indication. When one faces a patient with STEMI and MVD, the analysis of a heart team, where the scores are analyzed, the clinical status, the comorbidities, as well as the common sense should define the opportunity of the treatment of the non-culprit critical lesions.

4. Diabetes and multivessel disease

4.1 Introduction

DM is a global health problem; about 10% of adult patients will have the disease, and a quarter of all revascularized patients globally have DM [63]. However, patients with DM compared to nondiabetics have more MACCE and chronic heart failure. In addition, these patients have diffused and segmental disease, which puts them at greater risk of events regardless of the revascularization selected [64, 65]. PCI is limited by a higher rate of repeat revascularization and a worse clinical outcome in DM patients than with nondiabetic patients. CABG carries a greater morbidity, increased length of stay, and longer recovery times. However, both strategies have been improved during the last decade. In particular, the introduction of DES [66] has dramatically changed the landscape for PCI, with a significant reduction in the rate of restenosis especially the so-called second-generation stents that can reduce the gap [67]. The FREEDOM trial [68] demonstrated lower rates of major adverse cardiovascular events in patients with stable ischemic coronary disease who were assigned to CABG than with PCI using DES of first generation, at long-term follow-up. It is evident that this pathology carries a high atherogenic risk, and its current treatment is of surgical competence. Even so, we think that patients with a low ERACI score [17] are good candidates for PCI treatment, and the arrival of the new generation stents of Ultrathin-Strut DES [69] could reduce the gap that was created.

4.2 FREEDOM, critics, and main trials

This trial [68] has become the most important among patients with diabetes and type of revascularization as well as follow-up, which was carried out worldwide in 140 centers that included 1900 patients with DM with MVD who were randomized to PCI with DES from first generation or CABG and its long-term follow-up of at least 5 years. The primary end point was the combined mortality events of all causes, nonfatal MI, and stroke, such as MACCE. The MACCE was significantly in favor of the CABG (18.7% vs. 26.6%, $p < 0.005$), there was also a decrease in the mortality of all causes (10.9% vs. 16.9%, $p = 0.049$), the stroke was lower in the PCI group (2.4% vs. 5.2%, $p = 0.03$), and the revascularization of the treated vessel was highly significant in favor of the CABG almost three more times on the first year of follow-up. The nonfatal MI was almost double with the PCI group [68]. When the quality of life was evaluated, it was although slightly significantly better with surgery than with PCI; this is due to the amount of repeated revascularization. So, this study showed strong data and full impact on revascularization guidelines [70]. Also with respect to FREEDOM, a study of hospital costs was carried out; it was also favorable for surgical treatment vs. percutaneous treatment [71].

The study showed that the outcomes were significantly lower among patients randomized to CABG (18.7%) than patients randomized to PCI (26.6%) (**Figure 3A**). A closer look at how these rates were derived is warranted. A total of 1900 patients (953 in the PCI group and 947 in the CABG group) were enrolled

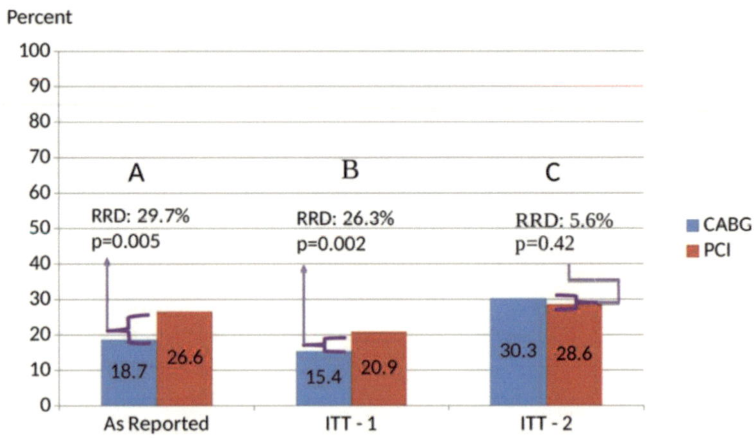

Figure 3.
A.B.C. FREEDOM trial results comparing ITT analyses. CABG, coronary arterial bypass graft surgery; ITT, intention-to-treat analysis; PCI, percutaneous coronary intervention. From "Critical appraisal of cardiology guidelines on revascularization: clinical practice" (David R Dobies and Kimberly R Barber).

and randomized. However, for the 5-year outcome rates, the denominator was 752 for PCI and 781 for CABG. These numbers are not the group totals but rather the number of patients remaining at risk at the end of the study. The number of events and the number remaining at risk are independent of each other. A basic occupant of a rate is that the subjects in the numerator are included in the denominator. The percentages the authors report are not rates; they are ratios and are very misleading. Calculating the events among the number randomized in each group results in a relative difference of 26% that is less significant than reported (**Figure 3B**). We would have more confidence in these recalculated rates if the study included all subjects in the denominator and accounted for outcomes on all subjects. They do not include the 214 (11.3%) patients lost to follow-up for whom we have no outcome data. This study also experienced a significant differential in attrition by group. The CABG group had twice the patients lost to follow-up (14.9%) as the PCI group did (7.7%). Revising the comparison by adding in the lost patients as events and calculating it with an intention-to-treat analysis (attributing events to the group of original assignment), we get a very different picture for the 5-year outcome (**Figure 3C**). The relative 5% difference is not significant ($p = 0.42$). This finding is in line with the 2-year composite outcomes in which the study authors observed no difference in outcome rates (13.0% vs. 11.9%, $p = 0.51$). The 5-year finding is significantly biased by the differential FREEDOM trial results comparing ITT analyses [72]. Other points of FREEDOM, which used first-generation stents that are currently discontinued, we remember presented a high rate of thrombosis stent [73]. Also in the trial a great geographical disparity was observed, since this difference marked by the study only was able to observe in the United States and the other centers in the randomization, and there were no significant differences outside of North American centers [68]. VA CARDS trial [74] is a study of veteran hospitals in the USA, in 22 centers, and included diabetic patients with MVD and 198 patients to be revascularized to PCI with DES or CABG with a 2-year follow-up. The primary end point of the study was the combined death events of all causes and nonfatal MI. The study was stopped early due to very slow recruitment by enrolling a quarter of the pre-established patients, which did not produce the power necessary for the evaluation of events. Within the study, it was observed that mortality in the 2-year PCI group reached a very high number up to 21% vs. 5% for CABG, while mortality was very high in the CABG group up to 15% compared with 6.2% for the PCI. This study was inconclusive. CARDia trial was a randomized study conducted in 22 centers in the United Kingdom and 2 centers in Ireland. Where Diabetic patients with MVD and patients with complex single lesion defined as ostial or proximal lesion of the anterior descending artery, which did not include LMCA between PCI or CABG, BMS was initially used, but when available the DES were used with the Axicimab adjuvant. A total of 510 patients were included, in which the primary end point was the MACCE, which included death of all causes, MI, and stroke. The study was non-inferior and with a 1-year follow-up. After 1 year the MACCE was 10.5% in the CABG group and 13% in the PCI group (HR, 1.25; 95% CI, 0.75–2.09; p = 0.39); the mortality of all the causes were the same in both groups of 3.2% (HR, 0.98; 95% CI, 0.37–2.6; p = 0.97). Although the study did not reach non-inferiority, it made the PCI as feasible [75].

4.3 Meta-analysis of MVD and DM

In this meta-analysis of the individual database of patients, where they analyzed 11 trials of patients with MVD followed in the long term, who were randomized to PCI or CABG, in the subgroup of patients with DM, it was observed that mortality was significantly higher in patients with PCI 15.7% than with CABG, which was 10.7% (p = 0.0001), while no differences were found among non-DM patients, 8.4% for CABG and 8.7% in the PCI group (p = 0.81) [43].

4.4 Our experience

In the ERACI III registry [76] which included 3 cohorts of 225 patients in each group with multiple MVD and PCI with DES, PCI with BMS, and patients with CABG, we analyzed the results of the subgroup of diabetic patients in each group at 3 years of follow-up. The incidence of MACCE at 3 years was significantly higher in diabetics than nondiabetics (RR, 0.81 [0.66–0.99]; p = 0.018). Higher rates of death and nonfatal AMI and a trend toward increased TVR, among others, were the principal determinants of increased MACCE. When stratified by treatment modality, MACCE rates among diabetics at 3 years were 36.2% in the DES arm, 43.6% in the BMS arm, and 30.8% in the CABG group (p = 0.49). There was a nonsignificant trend toward more death and nonfatal MI among diabetics in the ERACI III-DES cohort (19.1%) than in the BMS (12.8%) or CABG (15.4%) arms of ERACI II. Just as in the FREEDOM trial, the only stents used were the first-generation stents. Another limitation is that it was not a randomized trial, but they were two well-followed cohorts.

4.5 Can newer generation DES bridge the gap?

A total of 69 randomized trials that enrolled 24,015 diabetic patients with a total of 71,595 patient-years of follow-up satisfied our inclusion criteria. When compared with CABG (RR = 1.0), PCI with paclitaxel-eluting stent (RR = 1.57 [1.15–2.19]) or sirolimus-eluting stent (RR = 1.43 [1.06–1.97]) was associated with an increase in mortality. However, PCI with EES (RR = 1.11 [0.67–1.84]) was not associated with a statistically significant increase in mortality. In PCI with EES (RR = 1.31 [0.74–2.29]), the excess repeat revascularization was not statistically significant although the point estimate favored CABG. CABG was associated with numerically higher stroke. In patients with DM, evidence from indirect comparison shows similar mortality between CABG and PCI using EES. CABG was associated with numerically excess stroke and PCI with EES with numerically increased repeat revascularization [67].

4.6 Guidelines

Overall current evidence continues to favor CABG as the revascularization modality of choice for patients with diabetes and multivessel disease. When patients present with a comorbidity that increases surgical risk, the choice of revascularization method is best decided by multidisciplinary individualized risk assessment [20].

4.7 Conclusions

In this group of patients at high risk of diffuse coronary disease, there is evidence that patients with high scores are no doubt that surgery is the first option, although the only definitive evidence is FREEDOM despite its criticisms. Since the other studies could not be completed or did not show long-term follow-up, in patients with low scores, we believe that second-generation stents and perhaps new ultra-thin DES stents could shorten the gap between surgery events and angioplasty.

Author details

Juan Mieres* and Alfredo E. Rodríguez
Otamendi Hospital, Buenos Aires, Argentina

*Address all correspondence to: juanmieres@gmail.com

References

[1] Rodriguez AE, Baldi J, Fernández Pereira C, et al. Five-year follow-up of the argentine randomized trial of coronary angioplasty with stenting versus coronary bypass surgery in patients with multiple vessel disease (ERACI II). Journal of the American College of Cardiology. 2005;**46**(4):582-588

[2] Serruys PW, Morice MC, Kappetein AP, et al. Percutaneous coronary intervention versus coronary-artery bypass grafting for severe coronary artery disease. The New England Journal of Medicine. 2009;**360**(10):961-972

[3] Park SJ, Ahn JM, Kim YH, et al. Trial of everolimus-eluting stents or bypass surgery for coronary disease. The New England Journal of Medicine. 2015;**372**(13):1204-1212

[4] van Nunen LX, Zimmermann FM, Tonino PA, et al. Fractional flow reserve versus angiography for guidance of PCI in patients with multivessel coronary artery disease (FAME): 5-year follow-up of a randomised controlled trial. Lancet. 2015;**386**(10006):1853-1860

[5] Götberg M, Christiansen EH, Gudmundsdottir IJ, et al. Instantaneous wave-free ratio versus fractional flow reserve to guide PCI. The New England Journal of Medicine. 2017;**376**(19):1813-1823

[6] Al-Lamee R, Thompson D, Dehbi HM, et al. Percutaneous coronary intervention in stable angina (ORBITA): A double-blind, randomised controlled trial. Lancet. 2018;**391**(10115):31-40

[7] Thuesen AL, Riber LP, Veien KT, et al. Fractional flow reserve versus angiographically-guided coronary artery bypass grafting. Journal of the American College of Cardiology. 2018;**72**(22):2732-2743

[8] Farooq V, Brugaletta S, Serruys PW, et al. The SYNTAX score and SYNTAX-based clinical risk scores. Seminars in Thoracic and Cardiovascular Surgery. 2011;**23**:99-105

[9] Rodriguez AE, Fernandez-Pereira C, Mieres J, et al. Modifying angiographic syntax score according to PCI strategy: Lessons learnt from ERACI IV study. Cardiovascular Revascularization Medicine. 2015;**16**(7):418-420

[10] Negreiros de Andrade PJ, de Alencar Araripe Falcão JL, de Alencar Araripe Falcão B, et al. Stent versus coronary artery bypass surgery in multi-vessel and left Main coronary artery disease: A meta-analysis of randomized trials with subgroups evaluation. Arquivos Brasileiros de Cardiologia. 2019;**112**(5):511-523

[11] Kobayashi Y, Nam CW, Tonino PA, et al. The prognostic value of residual coronary stenoses after functionally complete revascularization. Journal of the American College of Cardiology. 2016;**67**:1701-1711

[12] Rodriguez A, Boullon F, Perez-Balino N, et al. Argentine randomized trial of percutaneous transluminal coronary angioplasty vs coronary artery bypass surgery in multi-vessel disease (ERACI): In hospital results and 1-year follow-up. Journal of the American College of Cardiology. 1993;**22**:1060-1067

[13] Rodriguez AE, Santaera O, Larribau M, et al. Second versus first drug eluting stents in complex lesions subsets: 3 years follow up of ERACI IV study. Minerva Cardioangiologica. 2017;**65**(1):81-90

[14] Rodriguez AE, Larribau M, Fernandez-Pereira C, et al. One-year follow-up results from the observational, multicenter, prospective, and controlled

registry: The WALTZ all-comers study. Clinical Medicine Insights: Cardiology. 2019;**13**:1179546819854059

[15] Mieres J, Lloberas J, Haeik C, et al. New cobalt-chromium stent design in the treatment of real world coronary artery disease: Rationality and study design of the all comers observational, multicenter and prospective WALTZ Registry. Revista Argentina de Cardioangiología. 2017;**1**:0012-0017

[16] Otsuka F, Finn AV, Kolodgie FD, et al. Pathology of second-generation everolimus-eluting stents versus first-generation sirolimus- and paclitaxel-eluting stents in humans. Circulation. 2014;**129**(2):211-223

[17] Shah T, Geleris JD, Zhong M, et al. Fractional flow reserve to guide surgical coronary revascularization. Journal of Thoracic Disease. 2017;**9**(Suppl 4):S317-S326

[18] Toth G, De Bruyne B, Casselman F, et al. Fractional flow reserve-guided versus angiography guided coronary artery bypass graft surgery. Circulation. 2013;**128**:1405-1411

[19] Fearon WF, Nishi T, De Bruyne B, et al. Clinical outcomes and cost-effectiveness of fractional flow reserve-guided percutaneous coronary intervention in patients with stable coronary artery disease: Three-year follow-up of the FAME 2 Trial (fractional flow reserve versus angiography for multivessel evaluation). Circulation. 2017;**031907**:117

[20] Neumann FJ, Sousa-Uva M, Ahlsson A, et al. 2018 ESC/EACTS guidelines on myocardial revascularization. European Heart Journal. 2019;**40**(2):87-165

[21] Patel MR, Calhoon JH, Dehmer GJ, et al. ACC/AATS/AHA/ASE/ASNC/SCAI/SCCT/STS 2017 appropriate use criteria for coronary revascularization in patients with stable ischemic heart disease: A report of the American College of Cardiology Appropriate use Criteria Task Force, American Association for Thoracic Surgery, American Heart Association, American Society of Echocardiography, American Society of Nuclear Cardiology, Society for Cardiovascular Angiography and Interventions, Society of Cardiovascular Computed Tomography, and Society of Thoracic Surgeons. Journal of Nuclear Cardiology. 2017;**24**(5):1759-1792

[22] ClinicalTrials.gov Identifier: NCT02894255

[23] ClinicalTrials.gov Identifier: NCT01034371

[24] Ragosta M, Dee S, Sarembock IJ, et al. Prevalence of unfavorable angiographic characteristics for percutaneous intervention in patients with unprotected left main coronary artery disease. Catheterization and Cardiovascular Interventions. 2006;**68**(3):357

[25] Capodanno D, Di Salvo ME, Seminara D, et al. Epidemiology and clinical impact of different anatomical phenotypes of the left main coronary artery. Heart and Vessels. 2011;**26**:138-144

[26] Takaro T, Peduzzi P, Detre KM, et al. Survival in subgroups of patients with left main coronary artery disease. Veterans administration cooperative study of surgery for coronary arterial occlusive disease. Circulation. 1982;**66**(1):14-22

[27] Morice M-C, Serruys PW, Kappetein AP, et al. Outcomes in patients with de novo left main disease treated with either percutaneous coronary intervention using paclitaxel-eluting stents or coronary artery bypass graft treatment in the synergy between percutaneous coronary

intervention with TAXUS and Cardiac Surgery (SYNTAX) Trial. Circulation. 2010;**121**:2645-2653

[28] Ahn JM, Roh JH, Kim YH, et al. Randomized trial of stents versus bypass surgery for left main coronary artery disease: 5-year outcomes of the PRECOMBAT study. Journal of the American College of Cardiology. 2015;**65**(20):2198-2206

[29] Buszman PE, Buszman PP, Banasiewicz-Szkróbka I, et al. Left main stenting in comparison with surgical revascularization: 10-year outcomes of the (left main coronary artery stenting) LE MANS Trial. JACC. Cardiovascular Interventions. 2016;**9**(4):318-327

[30] Mäkikallio T, Holm N, Lindsay M, et al. Percutaneous coronary angioplasty versus coronary artery bypass grafting in treatment of unprotected left main stenosis (NOBLE): A prospective, randomized, open-label, non-inferiority trial. Lancet. 2016;**388**(10061):2743-2752

[31] Stone GW, Sabik JF, Serruys PW, et al. Everolimus-eluting stents or bypass surgery for left main coronary artery disease. The New England Journal of Medicine. 2016;**375**(23):2223-2235

[32] Medina A, Suárez de Lezo J, Pan M, A new classification of coronary bifurcation lesions. Revista Española de Cardiología. 2006;**59**(2):183

[33] Chen SL, Xu B, Han YL, et al. Comparison of double kissing crush versus Culotte stenting for unprotected distal left main bifurcation lesions: Results from a multicenter, randomized, prospective DKCRUSH-III study. Journal of the American College of Cardiology. 2013;**61**:1482-1488

[34] Ali WE, Vaidya SR, Ejeh SU, Okoroafor KU. Meta-analysis study comparing percutaneous coronary intervention/drug eluting stent versus coronary artery bypass surgery of unprotected left main coronary artery disease: Clinical outcomes during short-term versus long-term (>1 year) follow-up. Medicine (Baltimore). 2018;**97**(7):e9909

[35] Xu B, Redfors B, Yang Y, et al. Impact of operator experience and volume on outcomes after left main coronary artery percutaneous coronary intervention. JACC. Cardiovascular Interventions. 2016;**9**:2086-2093

[36] Naganuma T, Chieffo A, Meliga E, et al. Long-term clinical outcomes after percutaneous coronary intervention for ostial/mid-shaft lesions versus distal bifurcation lesions in unprotected left main coronary artery: The DELTA Registry (drug-eluting stent for left main coronary artery disease): A multicenter registry evaluating percutaneous coronary intervention versus coronary artery bypass grafting for left main treatment. JACC. Cardiovascular Interventions. 2013;**6**:1242-1249

[37] Maeng M, Holm NR, Erglis A, et al. Long-term results after simple versus complex stenting of coronary artery bifurcation lesions: Nordic Bifurcation Study 5-year follow-up results. Journal of the American College of Cardiology. 2013;**62**:30-34

[38] Chen SL, Zhang JJ, Han Y, et al. Double kissing crush versus provisional stenting for left main distal bifurcation lesions: DKCRUSH-V randomized trial. Journal of the American College of Cardiology. 2017;**70**:2605-2617

[39] Kang SJ, Mintz GS, Kim WJ, et al. Changes in left main bifurcation geometry after a single-stent crossover technique: An intravascular ultrasound study using direct imaging of both the left anterior descending and the left circumflex coronary arteries before and after intervention. Circulation. Cardiovascular Interventions. 2011;**4**:355-361

[40] Kang SJ, Ahn JM, Song H, et al. Comprehensive intravascular ultrasound assessment of stent area and its impact on restenosis and adverse cardiac events in 403 patients with unprotected left main disease. Circulation. Cardiovascular Interventions. 2011;**4**:562-569

[41] IJsselmuiden AJJ, Zwaan EM, Oemrawsingh RM, et al. Appropriate use criteria for optical coherence tomography guidance in percutaneous coronary interventions recommendations of the working group of interventional cardiology of the Netherlands Society of Cardiology. Netherlands Heart Journal. 2018;**26**(10):473-483

[42] Hoye A. The proximal optimisation technique for intervention of coronary bifurcations. Interventional Cardiology. 2017;**12**(2):110-115

[43] Head SJ, Milojevic M, Daemen J, et al. Mortality after coronary artery bypass grafting versus percutaneous coronary intervention with stenting for coronary artery disease: A pooled analysis of individual patient data. Lancet. 2018;**391**:939-948

[44] ClinicalTrials.gov Identifier: NCT02303717

[45] ClinicalTrials.gov Identifier: NCT03544294

[46] Sorajja P, Gersh BJ, Cox DA, et al. Impact of multivessel disease on reperfusion success and clinical outcomes in patients undergoing primary percutaneous coronary intervention for acute myocardial infarction. European Heart Journal. 2007;**28**:1709-1716

[47] Kato K, Yonetsu T, Kim SJ, et al. Nonculprit plaques in patients with acute coronary syndromes have more vulnerable features compared with those with non-acute coronary syndromes: A 3-vessel optical coherence tomography study. Circulation. Cardiovascular Imaging. 2012;**5**:433-440

[48] Levine GN, Bates ER, Blankenship JC, et al. ACC/AHA/SCAI focused update on primary percutaneous coronary intervention for patients with st-elevation myocardial infarction: An update of the 2011 ACCF/AHA/SCAI guideline for percutaneous coronary intervention and the 2013 ACCF/AHA guideline for the management of ST Elevation myocardial infarction. Journal of the American College of Cardiology. 2015, 2016;**67**:1235-1250

[49] Wald DS, Morris JK, Wald NJ, et al. Randomized trial of preventive angioplasty in myocardial infarction. The New England Journal of Medicine. 2013;**369**:1115-1123

[50] Gershlick AH, Khan JN, Kelly DJ, et al. Randomized trial of complete versus lesion-only revascularization in patients undergoing primary percutaneous coronary intervention for STEMI and multivessel disease: The CvLPRIT trial. Journal of the American College of Cardiology. 2015;**65**:963-972

[51] Engstrøm T, Kelbæk H, Helqvist S, et al. Complete revascularisation versus treatment of the culprit lesion only in patients with ST-segment elevation myocardial infarction and multivessel disease (DANAMI-3—PRIMULTI): An open-label, randomised controlled trial. Lancet. 2015;**386**:665-671

[52] Smits PC, Abdel-Wahab M, Neumann FJ, Boxma-de Klerk BM, Lunde K, Schotborgh CE, et al. Fractional flow reserve-guided multivessel angioplasty in myocardial infarction. The New England Journal of Medicine. 2017;**376**:1234-1244

[53] Nagaraja V, Ooi SY, Nolan J, et al. Impact of incomplete percutaneous revascularization in patients with

multivessel coronary artery disease: A systematic review and meta-analysis. Journal of the American Heart Association. 2016;**5**(12). pii: e004598

[54] Hlinomaz O, Grouch L, Polokova L, et al. Multivessel coronary disease diagnosed at the time of primary PCI for STEMI: Complete revascularisation versus conservative strategy. PRAGUE-13 Trial Kardiologicka Revue. 2015;**17**:214-220

[55] Thiele H, Akin I, Sandri M, et al. One-year outcomes after PCI strategies in cardiogenic shock. The New England Journal of Medicine. 2018;**379**(18):1699-1710

[56] Park HW, Yoon CH, Kang SH, et al. Early- and late-term clinical outcome and their predictors in patients with ST-segment elevation myocardial infarction and non-ST segment elevation myocardial infarction. International Journal of Cardiology. 2013;**169**:254-261

[57] Jeong HC, Ahn JH, Kim MC, et al. A score for decision making during percutaneous coronary intervention in acute myocardial infarction patients with multivessel disease. The Korean Journal of Internal Medicine. 2019;**34**(2):324-334

[58] Elgendy IY, Mahmoud AN, Kumbhani DJ, et al. Complete or culprit-only revascularization for patients with multivessel coronary artery disease undergoing percutaneous coronary intervention: A pairwise and network meta-analysis of randomized trials. JACC: Cardiovascular Interventions. 2017;**10**:315-324

[59] Tamis-Holland JE, Suleiman A. The management of MVD in STEMI: The science and art of decision-making in STEMI. American College of Cardiology. 2018

[60] ClinicalTrials.gov Identifier NCT01740479

[61] ClinicalTrials.gov Identifier NCT02862119

[62] Rodriguez A, Bernardi V, Fernandez M, et al. In-hospital and late results of coronary stents versus conventional balloon angioplasty in acute myocardial infarction (GRAMI trial). Gianturco-Roubin in Acute Myocardial Infarction. American Journal of Cardiology. 1998;**81**:1286-1291

[63] Harris MI, Flegal KM, Cowie CC, et al. Prevalence of diabetes, impaired fasting glucose, and impaired glucose tolerance in U.S. adults. The Third National Health and Nutrition Examination Survey, 1988-1994. Diabetes Care. 1998;**21**:518-524

[64] Haffner SM, Lehto S, Ronnemaa T, et al. Mortality from coronary heart disease in subjects with type 2 diabetes and in non-diabetic subjects with and without prior myocardial infarction. The New England Journal of Medicine. 1998;**339**:229-234

[65] Natali A, Vichi A, Landi A, et al. Coronary atherosclerosis in type II diabetes: Angiographic findings and clinical outcomes. Diabetologia. 2000;**43**:632-641

[66] Jimenez-Quevedo P, Sabate M, Angiolillo DJ, et al. Long-term clinical benefit of sirolimus eluting stent implantation in diabetic patients with de novo coronary stenoses: Long-term results of the DIABETES trial. European Heart Journal. 2007;**28**:1946-1952

[67] Bangalore S, Toklu B, Feit F. Outcomes with coronary artery bypass graft surgery versus percutaneous coronary intervention for patients with diabetes mellitus: Can newer generation drug-eluting stents bridge the gap? Circulation. Cardiovascular Interventions. 2014;**7**(4):518-525

[68] Farkouh ME, Domanski M, Sleeper LA, et al. Strategies for multivessel revascularization in patients with diabetes. The New England Journal of Medicine. 2012;**367**(25):2375-2384

[69] Buiten RA, Ploumen EH, Zocca P, et al. Outcomes in patients treated with thin-strut, very thin-strut, or ultrathin-strut drug-eluting stents in small coronary vessels: A prespecified analysis of the randomized BIO-RESORT Trial. JAMA Cardiology. 2019;**4**(7):659-669

[70] Abdallah MS, Wang K, Magnuson EA, et al. Quality of life after PCI vs CABG among patients with diabetes and multivessel coronary artery disease: A randomized clinical trial. JAMA. 2013;**310**:1581-1590

[71] Magnuson EA, Farkouh ME, Fuster V, et al. Cost-effectiveness of percutaneous coronary intervention with drug eluting stents versus bypass surgery for patients with diabetes mellitus and multivessel coronary artery disease: Results from the FREEDOM trial. Circulation. 2013;**127**:820-831

[72] Dobies DR, Barber KR. Critical appraisal of cardiology guidelines on revascularisation: Clinical practice. Open Heart. 2018;**5**(1):e000779

[73] Rodríguez AE, Mieres J, Fernández-Pereira C, et al. Coronary stent thrombosis in the current drug-eluting stent era: Insights from the ERACI III trial. Journal of the American College of Cardiology. 2006;**47**(1):205-207

[74] Kamalesh M, Sharp TG, Tang XC, et al. Percutaneous coronary intervention versus coronary bypass surgery in United States veterans with diabetes. Journal of the American College of Cardiology. 2013;**61**(8):808-816

[75] Kapur A, Hall RJ, Malik IS, Qureshi AC, et al. Randomized comparison of percutaneous coronary intervention with coronary artery bypass grafting in diabetic patients. 1-year results of the CARDia (coronary artery revascularization in diabetes) trial. Journal of the American College of Cardiology. 2010;**55**(5):432-440

[76] Rodriguez AE, Maree AO, Mieres J, et al. Late loss of early benefit from drug-eluting stents when compared with bare-metal stents and coronary artery bypass surgery: 3 years follow-up of the ERACI III registry. European Heart Journal. 2007;**28**(17):2118-2125

[77] Morrison DA, Sethi G, Sacks J, et al. Percutaneous coronary intervention versus coronary artery bypass graft surgery for patients with medically refractory myocardial ischemia and risk factors for adverse outcomes with bypass: A multicenter, randomized trial. Investigators of the Department of Veterans Affairs Cooperative Study #385, the Angina With Extremely Serious Operative Mortality Evaluation (AWESOME). Journal of the American College of Cardiology. 2001;**38**(1):143-149

[78] Serruys PW, Unger F, Sousa JE, et al. Comparison of coronary-artery bypass surgery and stenting for the treatment of multivessel disease. Comparison of coronary-artery bypass surgery and stenting for the treatment of multivessel disease. The New England Journal of Medicine. 2001;**344**(15):1117-1124

[79] Booth J, Clayton T, Pepper J, et al. Randomized, controlled trial of coronary artery bypass surgery versus percutaneous coronary intervention in patients with multivessel coronary artery disease: Six-year follow-up from the Stent or Surgery Trial (SoS). Circulation. 2008;**118**(4):381-388

[80] Hueb W, Lopes N, Gersh BJ, et al. Ten-year follow-up survival of the medicine, angioplasty, or surgery study (MASS II): A randomized controlled

clinical trial of 3 therapeutic strategies for multivessel coronary artery disease. Circulation. 2010;**122**(10):949-957

[81] Boudriot E, Thiele H, Walther T, et al. Randomized comparison of percutaneous coronary intervention with sirolimus-eluting stents versus coronary artery bypass grafting in unprotected left main stem stenosis. Journal of the American College of Cardiology. 2011;**57**(5):538-545

Chapter 2

Evaluation of the Effect of Increased Arterial Stiffness on Ejection Performance and Pulmonary Arterial Pressure in Primary Mitral Regurgitation and Prediction of Ejection Fraction after Surgery: Analysis Using Wave Intensity

Kiyomi Niki and Motoaki Sugawara

Abstract

Mitral regurgitation (MR) is a common valvular disorder that has important health consequences. Surgical therapy is associated with reduced long-term mortality in elder patients. Several guidelines exist regarding when and in whom to perform mitral valve surgery, but they are controversial. It is essential to obtain preoperative indices that are promising for predicting postoperative left ventricular function and right ventricular pressure correctly. In aged MR patients, various hemodynamic conditions are presumed to be the causes of higher rate of mortality. In addition, aging causes increase in arterial stiffness. Therefore, it is also important to consider the effects of increased arterial stiffness on hemodynamics in MR. This review was written on the basis of our studies of wave intensity and will focus on the effects of increased arterial stiffness with a specific emphasis on wave intensity, which provides quantitative information about hemodynamic interaction between the ventricle and the arterial system.

Keywords: mitral regurgitation, arterial stiffness, wave intensity, surgical treatment, pulmonary hypertension

1. Introduction

A recent study reported that the rate of mortality among MR patients aged from 65 years upwards is higher compared with that expected among the general population, though the difference between younger MR patients and the general population is not significant [1]. Differences in age among the study groups are considered to yield different outcomes of a therapeutic strategy for treating severe

MR [2, 3]. The causes of the differences are considered to be reduced left atrial (LA) function and higher rate of complicated atrial fibrillation (AF) and increased ventricular myocardial stiffness in aged patients [2]. In addition to these factors, we consider that the effects of increased arterial stiffness, namely ventriculo-arterial coupling, are important.

The employed ultrasonic system provides arterial stiffness parameters and wave intensity (WI), which gives quantitative information about the dynamic behavior of the heart interacting with the vascular system [4–6]. Using indices obtained from measurements of wave intensity noninvasively, we analyzed the effects of changes in arterial stiffness on left ventricular (LV) performance and right ventricular pressure in MR and proposed a predictor of ejection fraction (EF) after surgery [7].

2. What is wave intensity?

Wave intensity (WI) is a hemodynamic index. It can be defined at any site in the circulatory system and evaluates the working condition of the heart interacting with the arterial system. WI is given by

$$WI = (dP/dt)(dU/dt), \tag{1}$$

where dP/dt and dU/dt are the time derivatives of pressure (P) and velocity (U) [6]. In a major artery of a healthy subject, two sharp positive peaks of WI are apparent during a cardiac cycle: wave 1 and wave 2 (**Figure 1**). Wave 1 occurs in early ejection and wave 2 occurs near end-ejection. The characteristics of these waves are theoretically described in the following way. According to the general theory of pulse waves traveling in an artery, the rates of changes in pressure and flow velocity at a fixed point caused by a forward wave and a backward (reflected) wave are related as follows, respectively:

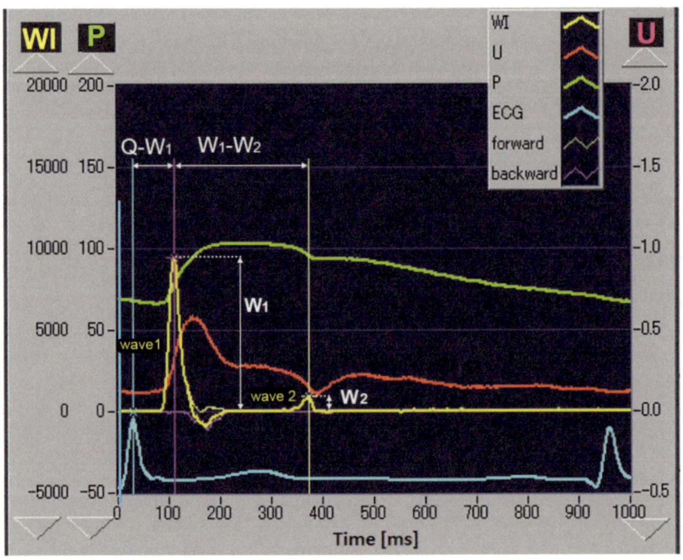

Figure 1.
Representative recordings of pressure P (mm Hg), blood flow velocity U (m/s), and calculated wave intensity WI (mm Hg m/s^3*) and electrocardiogram ECG obtained from a healthy subject. WI in a healthy subject shows two sharp peaks during a cardiac cycle, wave 1 and wave 2. Forward: forward wave component, backward: backward wave component.*

for a forward wave,

$$dPf/dt = \rho c dUf/dt \tag{2}$$

for a backward wave,

$$dPb/dt = -\rho c dUb/dt. \tag{3}$$

Here, dPf /dt and dUf/dt are the rates of changes in pressure and velocity caused by a forward wave, and dPb /dt and dUb/dt are those caused by a backward wave, respectively; ρ is the blood density, and c is the pulse wave velocity [8]. The actual measured rates of changes in pressure and velocity, dP/dt and dU/dt, are the sum of the rate of changes caused by a forward and a backward wave:

$$dP/dt = dPf/dt + dPb/dt, \tag{4}$$

$$dU/dt = dUf/dt + dUb/dt. \tag{5}$$

Using the above four equations, we can write WI as follows:

$$WI = (dP/dt)(dU/dt) = \left[(dPf/dt)^2 – (dPb/dt)^2\right]/\rho c = \rho c\left[(dUf/dt)^2 – (dUb/dt)^2\right]. \tag{6}$$

If WI > 0, the rates of changes caused by the forward wave, dPf/dt and dUf/dt, are greater than those caused by the backward wave, dPb/dt and dUb/dt, and vice versa. During the periods of wave 1 and wave 2, WI > 0 definitely, and dPb/dt and dUb/dt are nearly equal to zero [9]. The characteristics of these two positive waves are different. Wave 1 is associated with acceleration and an increase in pressure; thus it is a compression (pushing) wave. Wave 2 is associated with deceleration and a decrease in pressure and is therefore an expansion (suction) wave (**Figure 1**). The existence of suction wave near end-ejection was a surprising finding by Parker et al. [10], because it means that the left ventricle actively stops forward blood flow.

According to the description above, WI during the periods of wave 1 and wave 2 can be written as

$$WI = (dPf/dt)^2/\rho c. \tag{7}$$

Thus, the peak values of dPf/dt will give the peak values of WI, that is, W_1 and W_2. During the period of wave 1, the peak value of dPf/dt in the artery concerned is necessarily related to peak value of dPA/dt (peak dPA/dt), where PA is aortic pressure. It has been confirmed experimentally that peak dPA/dt is approximately equal to LV peak dP/dt [8]. Therefore, W_1 can be written as

$$W_1 \infty (\text{LV peak } dP/dt)^2/\rho c. \tag{8}$$

During the period of wave 2, it has been reported that negative peak dPf /dt is in proportion to the negative maximum value of ρcdUf /dt, that is, ρc times the maximum rate of deceleration (negative max dUf/dt) [11].

Therefore, W_2 can be written as

$$W_2 \infty (\rho c \text{ negative max } dUf/dt)^2/\rho c = \rho c \text{ (negtive max } dUf/dt)^2 \tag{9}$$

The interval between the Q wave of the ECG and W_1 (Q-W_1) and the interval between W_1 and W_2 (W_1–W_2) are used as surrogates for pre-ejection period and ejection time (**Figure 1**).

3. Noninvasive measurements of wave intensity and arterial stiffness

WI in major arteries is obtained noninvasively with a WI measuring system incorporated in ultrasonic diagnostic equipment, which measures arterial diameter-change waveform by echo tracking and blood flow velocity by color Doppler. Arterial diameter-change waveform is used as a surrogate for a blood pressure waveform [12] (see Appendix A.4). Henceforward, we will focus particularly on carotid arterial WI.

The WI measurement system also calculates the two arterial elastic moduli, stiffness parameter β [13] and pressure strain elastic modulus Ep, which are defined as follows:

$$\beta = \ln (Ps/Pd)/[(Ds - Dd)/Dd]$$

and

$$Ep = k(Ps - Pd)/[(Ds - Dd)/Dd],$$

where, Ps and Pd are systolic and diastolic pressures (mm Hg) and Ds and Dd are the maximum and minimum diameters (mm) of the carotid artery during a cardiac cycle, respectively. k = 0.133 (kPa/mm Hg), which is the factor for converting mmHg to kPa (10^3 N/m^2).

4. Relationship between wave intensity and arterial stiffness in healthy subjects

According to Eq. (8), W_1 is in inverse proportion to c. It is known that c increases with β [14]. Therefore, W_1 is expected to decrease with an increase in β if LV peak dP/dt and β change independently of each other. However, ventriculo-arterial couplings concerning the relation between changes in cardiac contractility (say peak dP/dt) and arterial stiffness (say β) have been reported. According to Kass D [15], age-related arterial stiffening is matched by ventricular systolic stiffening (increase in Emax), maintaining arterial-heart interaction age-independent. Indeed, our measurements in healthy subjects showed that changes in W_1 did not correlate with changes in β (**Figure 2a**).

5. Measurements of wave intensity in patients with MR and in healthy subjects

5.1 Population characteristics

We studied 98 consecutive patients with nonischemic chronic MR (60 men, age 52 ± 14 years) who underwent surgical treatment for MR and 98 age-matched and gender-matched healthy participants (60 men, age 52 ± 14 years) without any known cardiac disease, who were normotensive and had no history of serious noncardiac disease [7]. Informed consent was obtained from each subject, and the study protocol was approved by the ethics committee of Sakakibara Heart Institute. The characteristics of our study population are summarized in **Table 1**. There were no significant differences in hemodynamic data between the MR group and the healthy group except systolic and diastolic pressures, which were lower in the MR (**Table 2**). The etiologies of MR were as follows. Fibroelastic degeneration (n = 83), billowing leaflets

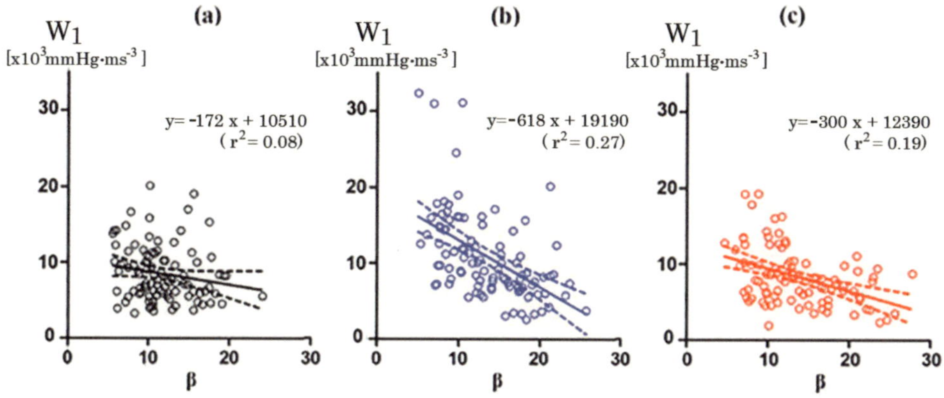

Figure 2.
Relations between W1 and β in (a) healthy control group, (b) MR group before surgery, and (c) MR group after surgery. The solid lines show the regression line. The slope of the regression line in (a) does not significantly deviate from zero (p = 0.08). The slope of the regression line in (b) deviates from zero significantly (p < 0.0001). The difference in the slope of regression line between (a) and (c) is not significant (p = 0.65).

	MR subjects	Healthy control
Number	98	98
Age (years)	52 ± 14	52 ± 14
Sex (men/women)	60/38	60/38
Height (m)	1.65 ± 0.10	1.64 ± 0.10
Weight (kg)	61 ± 12	61 ± 11
BSA (m^2)]	1.66 ± 0.20	1.67 ± 0.18

MR, mitral regurgitation; BSA, body surface area.

Table 1.
Clinical characteristics [7].

(n = 2), Barlow's disease (n = 4), healed infective endocarditis (n = 5), rheumatism (n = 3), or cleft (n = 1). The surgical therapies (valve repair in 90 patients and replacement in 8 patients) were performed successfully in all patients.

Representative recordings of WI before and after surgery are shown in **Figure 3**. β was highly significantly correlated with age both in the MR group and the healthy group (r = 0.74, p < 0.001; r = 0.70, P < 0.001, respectively). W_1 was not correlated with β in the healthy group (goodness of fit R^2 = 0.02, p = 0.08) (**Figure 2a**) as mentioned above.

5.2 Effects of increased arterial stiffness on wave intensity in MR before and after surgery

The MR group before surgery showed higher W_1, and unlike the healthy group, W_1 was correlated with β in MR group before surgery (R^2 = 0.26, p < 0.0001) (**Figure 2b**). To elucidate this relationship, it is necessary to give full consideration to the particular ejection dynamics of MR, that is, simultaneous ejection to the aorta and the left atrium.

Regurgitation (ejection to the left atrium) is accompanied by increase in preload (LVEDVI), which enhances LV peak dP/dt, hence W_1. Contrary to this, increase in β is reported to be associated with a decrease in LV end-diastolic chamber diameter [16], which decreases preload, hence W_1. Wohlfahrt et al. [17] also reported that

	MR		Healthy control
	Before surgery	After surgery	
W_1 ($\times 10^3$mm Hg · m/s^3)	$10.7 \pm 5.7^{*}$	$8.3 \pm 3.7^{\xi}$	$8.5 \pm 3.6^{\xi}$
W_2 ($\times 10^3$mm Hg · m/s^3)	$0.8 \pm 0.6^{**}$	$2.4 \pm 1.0^{*\xi\xi}$	$1.9 \pm 0.8^{\xi\xi}$
(Q-W_1)st (ms)	171 ± 16	$189 \pm 22^{**\xi\xi}$	167 ± 10
(W_1-W_2)st (ms)	$330 \pm 24^{**}$	$320 \pm 23^{**\xi}$	$357 \pm 15^{\xi\xi}$
β	$13.6 \pm 4.8^{*}$	$13.7 \pm 5.2^{*}$	$11.6 \pm 3.8^{\xi}$
Ep (kPa)	149 ± 58	141 ± 58	142 ± 50
Ps (mm Hg)	$110 \pm 11^{**}$	$102 \pm 12^{**\xi\xi}$	$118 \pm 12^{\xi\xi}$
Pd (mm Hg)	$59 \pm 10^{**}$	$56 \pm 8^{**\xi}$	$69 \pm 9^{\xi\xi}$
HR (bpm)	65 ± 10	$71 \pm 12^{*\xi}$	64 ± 10

WI indices (W_1, W_2, Q-W_1, and W_1-W_2) are the same as ***Figure 1****; suffix st, see text; β, stiffness parameter; Ep, pressure strain elastic modulus; Ps, systolic blood pressure; Pd, diastolic blood pressure; HR, heart rate.*
*vs. healthy subjects ($^{*}p < 0.05$, $^{**}p < 0.001$); $^{\xi}$ vs. before surgery ($^{\xi}p < 0.05$, $^{\xi\xi}p < 0.001$).

Table 2.
WI indices and arterial stiffness [7].

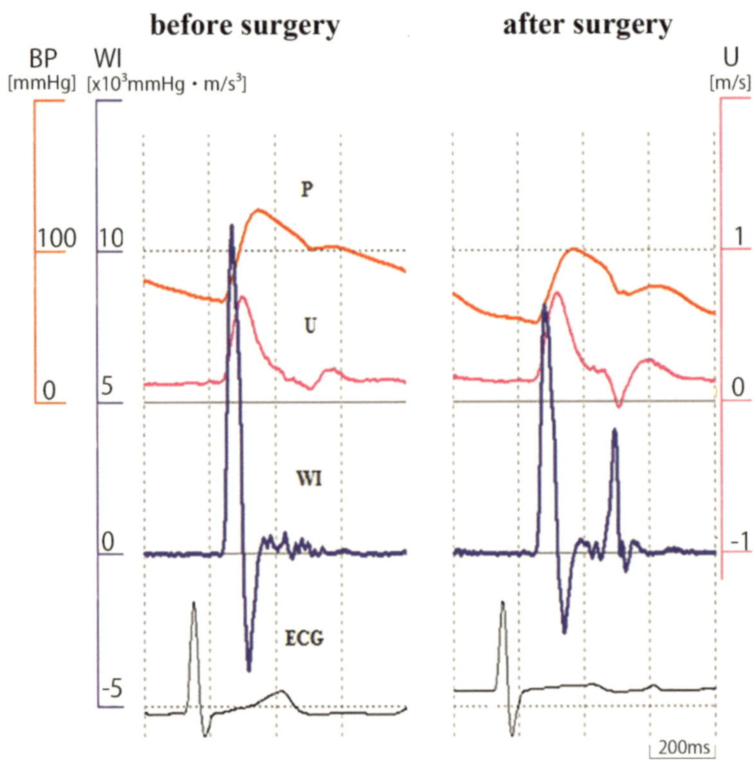

Figure 3.
Representative recordings of wave intensity in an MR subject before and after surgery. After the surgery, W1 is decreased and W2 is increased compared with before surgery. BP is blood pressure.

loss of arterial compliance plays an important role in LV stiffening during diastole. Indeed in our study, increase in β was associated with decrease in LVEDVI both before and after surgery (**Table 3**). Therefore, the diastolic LV stiffening associated with increase in β is considered to cause a decrease in W_1 in MR with higher β.

Increase in β is also associated with an increase in RegF/EOR (**Table 3**), that is, the leakage from the pressure chamber. As a result, the ventricular systolic stiffening and increase in preload by regurgitation did not work effectively in augmenting the initial pressure rise (LV peak dP/dt) in MR with higher β. Therefore, a compensatory increase in W_1 was observed only in MR with lower β and contraction preserved hearts. In other words, higher W_1 in MR is observed only in young population. On the whole in MR, W_1 was higher for lower β and lower for higher β, which made the negative slope of the regression line of W_1 on β significantly steep (**Figure 2b**). After the surgery, W_1 decreased. Though the correlation was still significant ($R^2 = 0.18$, $p = 0.0004$), the slope of the regression line of W_1 on β became gentle (**Figure 2c**), and the difference in the slope between the healthy subjects and MR groups became not significant ($p = 0.65$), which suggests that the steeper regression of W_1 on β was caused by regurgitation. There was no change in β after surgery.

5.3 Other wave intensity indices and arterial stiffness in MR patients and healthy subjects

The values of the WI indices in the MR before and after surgery and in the healthy subjects are summarized in **Table 2**. W_2 in MR was significantly reduced and negatively correlated with ERO ($r = 0.37$, $p < 0.001$). W_2 is an expansion (suction) wave produced by the heart, when blood flows out of the left ventricle into the aorta under its own momentum, which causes a rapid decline in left

	Before surgery		**After surgery**	
		r		**r**
LVEDVI (ml/m^2)	89 ± 20	−0.30^{ξ}	61 ± 16**	−0.22^{ξ}
LVESVI (ml/m^2)	32 ± 10	−0.26^{ξ}	29 ± 12**	−0.16
EF (%)	64 ± 7	0.11	54 ± 9**	0.08
LAVI (ml/m^2)	78 ± 27	0.13	51 ± 17**	0.13
RVSP (mm Hg)	39 ± 15	0.36^{ξξ}	26 ± 6**	0.03
E/A	2.03 ± 0.77	−0.25^{ξ}	1.55 ± 0.77**	−0.26^{ξ}
E/e′	14.1 ± 6.0	0.43^{ξξ}	19.4 ± 6.9**	0.02
e′	9.7 ± 2.7	−0.57^{ξξ}	6.4 ± 1.8**	−0.21^{ξ}
ERO (cm^2)	0.48 ± 0.17	−0.11		
RegV (ml)	69 ± 16	−0.19		
RegF (%)	55 ± 8	0.11		
RegV/ERO (ml/cm^2)	152 ± 35	−0.02		
RegF/ERO (%/cm^2)	124 ± 34	0.23 ^{ξ}		
Reduction rate of RVSP (%)			25.6 ± 29.0	0.42^{ξ}
$(Q\text{-}W_1)st$ (ms)	171 ± 16	−0.14	189 ± 22	0.01

LVED(S)VI, left ventricular end-diastolic (systolic) volume index; EF, ejection fraction; LAVI, left atrial volume index; RVSP, right ventricular systolic pressure; ERO, effective regurgitant orifice area; RegV, regurgitant volume; RegF, regurgitant fraction (RegV / total LV stroke volume); WI index ($Q\text{-}W_1$) is the same as ***Figure 1****; suffix st, see text; β, stiffness parameter; reduction rate of RVSP, (RVSP before surgery − RVSP after surgery)/RVSP before surgery × 100; comparison between before and after surgery *$p < 0.05$, **$p < 0.001$; r, correlation with β $^{ξ}p < 0.05$, $^{ξξ}p < 0.001$.*

Table 3.
Echocardiographic data and $(Q\text{-}W_1)st$ before and after surgery in mitral regurgitation and correlation with β [7].

ventricular pressure and a rapid increase in the maximum rate of deceleration (negative max dUf/dt) in the aorta (hence in the artery concerned) near end-ejection [5, 6, 18]. Thus, we obtained Eq. (9) above. In MR before surgery, negative max dUf /dt is very small or sometimes nearly zero as shown in **Figure 3**, left, which causes a reduction in W_2. After the repair of regurgitation, negative max dUf/dt recovers and sometimes becomes greater than the normal values as shown in **Figure 3**, right, which causes a recovery in W_2.

Q-W_1 and W_1-W_2 were temporal indices of WI, and the dependency of Q-W_1 and W_1-W_2 on heart rate was observed in the healthy group (Q-W_1 = −0.51 HR +167, $r = 0.44$, $p < 0.0001$; W_1-W_2 = −1.33 HR + 358, $r = 0.68$, $p < 0.0001$). Therefore, based on the method by Lewis et al. [19], the standardized indices were defined as follows:

$$(Q - W_1)st = 0.51\ HR + Q - W_1,$$

and

$$(W_1 - W_2)st = 1.33\ HR + W_1 - W_2,$$

which were expected not to depend on HR in the healthy subjects and MR group before surgery. As compared with the healthy subjects, the MR group before surgery showed shorter (W_1-W_2)st (**Table 2**). The stiffness parameter β but not Ep was higher in the MR group (see Appendix A.3).

6. Clinical application of wave intensity for planning the treatment of MR

6.1 Effects of the changes in arterial stiffness on pulmonary hypertension before and after surgery

Pulmonary hypertension (PH) is one of the conclusive factors of surgical indication in MR, though the PH in MR emerges through multifactorial processes. In our study, patients with EF lower than 40% were not included. Therefore, we do not consider that the major cause of PH was left ventricular systolic failure. The results of linear univariate and following stepwise multivariate regression analyses to identify predictor variables before surgery to determine RVSP showed that ERO, β, and LAVI were independent predictor variables (**Table 4**). Increase in β, hence increase in c, increases LV afterload during initial ejection (characteristic impedance ρc [20]). In MR during ejection, there is a pressure gradient between the left ventricle and the left atrium, which is in proportion to the square of regurgitation velocity. In other words, LV pressure during ejection is paradoxically supported by regurgitation velocity toward the left atrium. Therefore, for the left ventricle to eject the blood against higher ρc, higher regurgitation velocity, hence greater regurgitation volume, is required. This makes LAVI in MR greater. In fact, the ratio of regurgitant fraction to ERO (Reg F ratio) increased with an increase in β ($r = 0.23$, $p = 0.027$) (**Table 3**). This result indicates that increased arterial stiffness exacerbates pulmonary hypertension, which will recover immediately after correction of MR (cessation of regurgitation). There was a strong correlation between RVSP and β before surgery, but this correlation disappeared after surgery (**Table 3**). The reduction rate of RVSP by surgery increased with increase in β (**Table 3**). This suggests that the surgical repair of MR caused more beneficial effect of improving PH in MR with higher β than with lower β. Surgical therapy was

	Univariate analysis		**Multivariate analysis $R^2 = 0.34$ (adjusted $R^2 = 0.31$, $p < 0.001$)**		
Variables before surgery	**r**	**p**	**Beta**	**p**	**VIF**
W_1	−0.21	0.039	−0.11	0.283	1.381
W_2	0.05	0.658			
β	0.36	< 0.001	0.35	< 0.001	1.025
$(Q\text{-}W_1)st$	−0.08	0.44			
LVEDVI	0.15	0.145			
LVESVI	0.14	0.169			
EF	−0.02	0.853			
LAVI	0.31	0.003	0.2	0.031	1.062
E/A	0.08	0.459			
e′	−0.29	0.004	−0.17	0.114	1.62
ERO	0.36	< 0.001	0.37	< 0.001	1.039

*WI indices (W_1, W_2, and $Q\text{-}W_1$) are the same as **Figure 1**; suffix st, see text; LVED(S)VI, left ventricular end-diastolic (systolic) volume index; EF, ejection fraction; LAVI, left atrial volume index; ERO, effective regurgitant orifice area; Beta, standardized coefficients; VIF, variance inflation factor.*

Table 4.
Results of univariate and multivariate linear regression analyses for determinants of right ventricular systolic pressure before surgery [7].

reported to improve long-term mortality in older patients [1]. However, the long-term prognosis of surgically treated MR patients with PH, which included more aged patients, was still worse than that of patients without PH. According to Murashita et al. [21], preoperative PH disappeared after surgery in degenerative MR patients, and the most important cause of cardiovascular death after surgery was stroke, and most of patients who had recurrence of PH suffered from AF, which suggested that recurrent PH after surgery was caused by different pathophysiology due to PH before surgery.

6.2 Usefulness of wave intensity indices in predicting EF after surgery

As a surrogate for pre-ejection time, $(Q\text{-}W_1)st$ has the potential for properly evaluating cardiac performance. $Q\text{-}W_1$ is the sum of PEP, the transit time of the pulse wave from the left ventricle to the carotid artery and the time from the beginning of ejection to the peak of wave 1. PEP is an old concept, but its high sensitivity and reproducibility are still useful in indicating reduced performance of the myocardium in its early stage. Therefore, the change in $(Q\text{-}W_1)st$ also reflects the changes in myocardial properties due to remodeling. The statistical analysis using stepwise multivariate regression in our study showed that EF and $(Q\text{-}W_1)st$ before surgery are selected predictor variables for the response variable EF after surgery (**Table 5**). $(Q\text{-}W_1)st$ was an index with higher specificity to predict EF after surgery than the preoperative EF. The receiver-operator characteristic (ROC) curve was constructed to define optimal cut-off in $(Q\text{-}W_1)st$ to predict low EF after surgery (<50%) using the guideline criteria outlined above. The selected cut-off value for low EF was 180 ms, which gave a sensitivity of 57% and a specificity of 87% for predicting EF after surgery lower than 50% (area under ROC 0.72, p = 0.001)

	Univariate analysis		Multivariate analysis $R^2 = 0.34$ (adjusted $R^2 = 0.32$, $p < 0.001$)		
Variables before surgery	**r**	**p**	**Beta**	**p**	**VIF**
Age	0.27	0.008	−0.04	0.657	1.193
W_1	0.08	0.449			
W_2	−0.15	0.154			
β	0.02	0.832			
$(Q\text{-}W_1)$st	−0.52	< 0.001	−0.39	< 0.001	1.274
LVEDVI	−0.27	0.007	−0.14	0.106	1.097
EF	0.47	< 0.001	0.28	0.004	1.274
LAVI	−0.1	0.353			
E/A	−0.21	0.041	−0.14	0.101	1.017
e′	0.02	0.862			
RVSP	−0.1	0.338			

WI indices (W_1, W_2, and Q-W_1) are the same as ***Figure 1****; suffix st, see text; LVEDVI, left ventricular end-diastolic volume index; EF, ejection fraction; LAVI, left atrial volume index; RVSP, right ventricular systolic pressure; Beta, standardized coefficients; VIF, variance inflation factor.*

Table 5.
Results of univariate and multivariate linear regression analyses for determinants of EF after surgery [7].

(**Figure 4a**). The cut-off value of EF before surgery, 60%, gave a sensitivity of 81% and a specificity of 57% for predicting reduced EF after surgery (< 50%) (area under ROC 0.73, p = 0.001) (**Figure 4b**). Furthermore, among the subgroup with EF before surgery <60% (n = 26), the cut-off value of $(Q\text{-}W_1)$st, 180 ms, gave a sensitivity of 81% and a specificity of 90% for predicting reduced EF after surgery (< 50%) (area under ROC 0.73, p < 0.001) (**Figure 4c**).

EF before surgery is still one of the valuable parameters to predict survival rate after surgical treatment and it is expected that the best outcome is obtained when surgical treatment is taken into account before EF reduces to a level under 60% [22]. Asymptomatic stage of chronic MR patients often lasts for a long time, and such patients are usually reluctant to undergo surgery. Such situation seems to be more common in patients with lower arterial stiffness, because PH occurs less

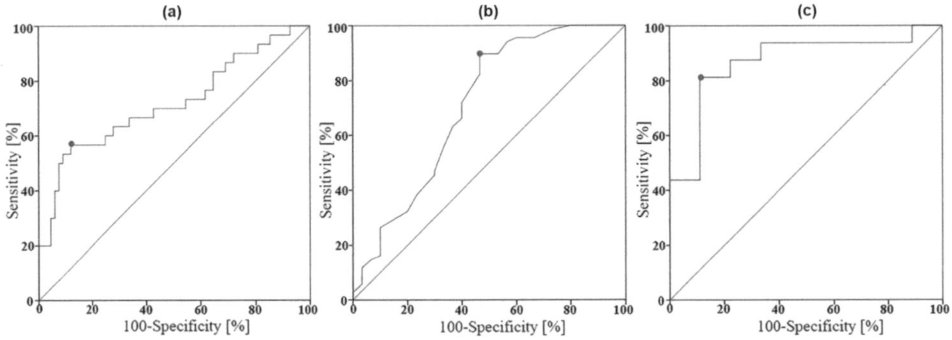

Figure 4.
Receiver-operator characteristic curves and selected combinations of sensitivity and specificity (red dots) to predict EF after surgery <50%. (a) Cut-off value of (Q-W1)st before surgery = 180 ms, (b) cut-off value of EF before surgery = 60%, and (c) cut-off value of (Q-W1)st before surgery = 180 ms in the subgroup of patients with EF before surgery <60% (from [7]).

frequently compared with subjects with higher arterial stiffness. Therefore, it is desirable to convince MR patients, who have signs of the beginning of deterioration of myocardial function, of the benefits of surgical treatment. By using both indices ($(Q\text{-}W_1)st > 180$ ms and EF $< 60\%$), prediction of low EF after surgery with higher sensitivity and specificity is possible.

7. Conclusions

Increased arterial stiffness affects forward flow and exacerbates pulmonary hypertension in MR. Since arterial stiffness is not reduced by vasodilator or diuretics, such medication is not so efficient at improving pulmonary hypertension caused by increased arterial stiffness, while surgical correction of MR improves the pulmonary hypertension markedly. In a paradoxical manner, pulmonary hypertension in subjects with lower arterial stiffness is caused by depressed heart, which would be difficult to recover after surgery. Prolonged (Q-W1)st indicates that the heart reached a preliminary stage in remodeling that would be irreversible even after surgery.

Conflict of interest

The authors declare no conflict of interest.

A. Appendix

A.1 Echocardiographic evaluation

In this study, echocardiographic evaluation was performed in MR subjects before and after surgery using an echo machine (SONOS 7500; Philips) [23]. LV and left atrial volume (LAV) were determined using the modified Simpson's method. LAV was measured at the end-systole just before the mitral valve opening, and LV and LA volume indices, which were divided by the body surface area, were obtained. Right ventricular systolic pressure (RVSP) was obtained by adding the systolic tricuspid pressure gradient calculated by the modified Bernoulli equation and right atrial pressure [24]. Transmitral flow was assessed using pulsed Doppler by placing the sample volume at the level of leaflet tips, and early filling (E) and atrial contraction filling (A) velocities were measured. Tissue Doppler velocity of the mitral annulus in early diastole (e') was also measured. MR severity was quantified as averaged effective regurgitant orifice area (ERO) obtained by the Doppler volumetric method [25].

A.2 Statistical analysis

As for statistical analysis, comparisons among groups were performed by Student's t test or one way analyses of variance, followed by Bonferroni test when necessary. The relationships between WI indices and β were evaluated by correlation and regression analysis. Univariate regression analyses were performed for the data relating pulmonary hypertension before surgery to the variables measured before surgery and for the data relating EF after surgery to the variables measured before surgery. Then, the variables that were correlated with RVSP before surgery and EF after surgery ($p \leq 0.1$) were entered into stepwise multivariate regression models. To obtain the threshold value of predictor variable separating a clinical diagnosis that EF after surgery≥50% from one that EF after surgery <50%, the ROC curves were created, and the optimal combinations of sensitivity and specificity were chosen. A p value <0.05 was set for statistical significance.

A.3 Proper index of arterial stiffness

β is considered not to depend on pressure, while Ep decreases with a decrease in pressure. Most of the severe MR patients with hypertension were medicated with antihypertensive drugs. Therefore, in our study, systolic pressure in MR was lower than that in the healthy subject group, and there was no difference in Ep between the two groups. However, β was higher in MR. We consider that the increase in β was not caused by MR but caused by the history of hypertension. Actually, 38% of the patients were diagnosed as hypertension and medicated. Thus, β is suitable to evaluate arterial stiffness in low pressure subjects.

A.4 Use of upper arm blood pressure for calibration of carotid arterial pressure waveform

The use of upper arm pressure for calibrating carotid arterial pressure (diameter) might be criticized. In young adults, the peak pressure in the upper arm is higher than the peak pressures in central predominantly elastic arteries such as the aorta and the carotid artery (amplification). The peak pressures in central arteries increase with age due to increase in arterial stiffness by aging (late systolic peaking). In contrast, there is little or no consistent change in stiffness of the brachial or radial arteries and little change in the peak pressure in the upper arm. Therefore, the difference between central peak pressures and upper arm pressure becomes less significant in the elderly [20]. Ohte et al. [26] reported that the systematic difference between those in 82 patients (age 64.3 ± 9.4 years) remained within the practical range.

A.5 Where to set the positions for echo tracking to measure arterial diameter change waveforms

The relative change in arterial diameter, (Ds − Dd)/Dd, measured in an inner layer (e.g., intima) is greater than that measured in an outer layer (e.g., adventitia) due to incompressibility of the arterial wall. Therefore, β is smaller for an inner layer than for an outer layer. In some institutions, β is obtained by echo tracking the intima and in other institutions by echo tracking the adventitia. Then the obtained value of β for a patient may vary with the institution. We obtained β by setting the positions for echo tracking in the adventitia for the following reasons: 1) it is easier to obtain stable tracking. 2) The PWV calculated from the β obtained from the adventitia agrees well with the PWV obtained by a different method [14].

Author details

Kiyomi Niki[1]* and Motoaki Sugawara[1,2]

1 Tokyo Women's Medical University, Tokyo, Japan

2 Himeji Dokkyo University, Himeji, Japan

*Address all correspondence to: nikiwi@cosmos.ocn.ne.jp

References

[1] Avierinos J-F, Tribouilloy C, Grigioni F, Suri R, Barbieri A, Michelena HI, et al. Impact of ageing on presentation and outcome of mitral regurgitation due to flail leaflet: A multicentre international study. European Heart Journal. 2013;**34**(33):2600-2609

[2] Avierinos JF. Mitral regurgitation due to mitral valve prolapse: Four decades of controversies. Archives of Cardiovascular Diseases. 2014;**107**(3): 145-148

[3] Rosenhek R, Rader F, Klaar U, Gabriel H, Krejc M, Kalbeck D, et al. Outcome of watchful waiting in asymptomatic severe mitral regurgitation. Circulation. 2006; **113**(18):2238-2244

[4] Parker KH, Jones CJH. Forward and backward running waves in the arteries: Analysis using the method of characteristics. ASME. Journal of Biomechanical Engineering. 1990;**112**: 322-326

[5] Ramsey MW, Sugawara M. Arterial wave intensity and ventriculoarterial interaction. Heart and Vessels. 1997;**12** (Suppl):128-134

[6] Sugawara M, Niki K, Ohte N, Okada T, Harada A. Clinical usefulness of wave intensity analysis. Medical & Biological Engineering & Computing. 2009;**47**(2):197-206

[7] Niki K, Sugawara M, Kayanuma H, Takamisawa I, Watanabe H, Mahara K, et al. Associations of increased arterial stiffness with left ventricular ejection performance and right ventricular systolic pressure in mitral regurgitation before and after surgery: Wave intensity analysis. IJC Heart and Vasculature. 2017;**16**:7-13

[8] Sugawara M, Senda S, Katayama H, Masugata H, Nishiya T, Matsuo H. Noninvasive estimation of left ventricular max (dP/dt) from aortic flow acceleration and pulse wave velocity. Echocardiography. 1994;**11**(4):377-384

[9] Niki K, Sugawara M, Uchida K, Tanaka R, Tanimoto K, Imamura H, et al. A noninvasive method of measuring wave intensity, a new hemodynamic index: Application to the carotid artery in patients with mitral regurgitation before and after surgery. Heart and Vessels. 1999;**14**(6):263-271

[10] Parker KH, Jones CJH, Dawson JR, Gibson DG. What stops the flow of blood from the heart? Heart and Vessels. 1988;**4**:241-245

[11] Sugawara M, Uchida K, Kondoh Y, Magosaki N, Niki K, Jones CJH, et al. Aortic blood momentum - the more the better for the ejecting heart in vivo? Cardiovascular Research. 1997;**33**: 433-446

[12] Niki K, Sugawara M, Chang D, Harada A, Okada T, Sakai R, et al. A new noninvasive measurement system for wave intensity: Evaluation of carotid arterial wave intensity and reproducibility. Heart and Vessels. 2002;**17**(1):12-21

[13] Kawasaki T, Sasayama S, Yagi S-I, Asakawa T, Hirai T. Non-invasive assessment of the age related changes in stiffness of major branches of the human arteries. Cardiovascular Research. 1987;**21**(9):678-687

[14] Harada A, Okada T, Niki K, Chang D, Sugawara M. On-line noninvasive one-point measurements of pulse wave velocity. Heart and Vessels. 2002;**17**(2):61-68

[15] Kass DA. Age-related changes in venticular–arterial coupling: Pathophysiologic implications. Heart Failure Reviews. 2002;**7**(1):51-62

[16] Roman MJ, Ganau A, Saba PS, Pini R, Pickering TG, Devereux RB. Impact of arterial stiffening on left ventricular structure. Hypertension. 2000;**36**(4):489-494

[17] Wohlfahrt P, Redfield MM, Melenovsky V, Lopez-Jimenez F, Rodeheffer RJ, Borlaug BA. Impact of chronic changes in arterial compliance and resistance on left ventricular ageing in humans. European Journal of Heart Failure. 2015;**17**(1):27-34

[18] Jones CJH, Sugawara M, Davies RH, Kondoh Y, Uchida K, Parker KH. Arterial wave intensity: Physical meaning and physiological significance. In: Hosoda S, Yaginuma T, Sugawara M, Taylor MG, Caro CG, editors. Recent Progress in Cardiovascular Mechanics: Chur Harwood Academic Publishers; 1994. pp. 129-148

[19] Lewis RP, Rittogers S, Froester W, Boudoulas H. A clitical review of the systolic time intervals. Circulation. 1977; **56**(2):146-158

[20] Nichols W, O'Rourke M. McDonald's blood flow in arteries. In: Theoretical, Experimental and Clinical Principles. 5th ed. London: Hodder Arnold; 2005. p. 265

[21] Murashita T, Okada Y, Kanemitsu H, Fukunaga N, Konishi Y, Nakamura K, et al. Feasibility and efficacy of mitral valve repair for degenerative mitral regurgitation in the elderly. Annals of Thoracic and Cardiovascular Surgery. 2014;**20**(6): 1001-1007

[22] Tribouilloy C, Rusinaru D, Grigioni F, Michelena HI, Vanoverschelde J-L, Avierinos J-F, et al. Long-term mortality associated with left ventricular dysfunction in mitral regurgitation due to flail leaflets a multicenter analysis. Circulation: Cardiovascular Imaging. 2014;**7**(2): 363-370

[23] Lang RM, Bierig M, Devereux RB, Flachskampf FA, Foster E, Pellikka PA, et al. Recommendations for chamber quantification: A report from the American Society of Echocardiography's guidelines and standards committee and the chamber quantification writing group, developed in conjunction with the European Association of Echocardiography, a branch of the European Society of Cardiology. Journal of the American Society of Echocardiography. 2005;**18**(12): 1440-1463

[24] Kircher BJ, Himelman RB, Schiller NB. Noninvasive estimation of right atrial pressure from the inspiratory collapse of the inferior vena cava. The American Journal of Cardiology. 1990; **66**(4):493-496

[25] Zoghbi W. Recommendations for evaluation of the severity of native valvular regurgitation with two-dimensional and doppler echocardiography. Journal of the American Society of Echocardiography. 2003;**16**(7):777-802

[26] Ohte N, Saeki T, Miyabe H, Sakata S, Mukai S, Hayano J, et al. Relationship between blood pressure obtained from the upper arm with a cuff-type sphygmomanometer and central blood pressure measured with a catheter-tipped micromanometer. Heart and Vessels. 2007;**22**(6):410-415

Chapter 3

Antiplatelet Therapy after Coronary Artery Bypass Graft Surgery, Inconsistency of Clinical Practice and Clinical Significance of Proven Resistance to Antiplatelet Agents

Ivana Sopek Merkas, Nenad Lakusic, Krunoslav Fuckar, Dusko Cerovec and Kristina Maric Besic

Abstract

Antiplatelet therapy is a very important part of medical therapy for patients after acute coronary syndrome (ACS) as well as in a stable coronary artery disease (CAD). The use of antiplatelet therapy after coronary artery bypass graft surgery (CABG) still is a controversial theme in daily clinical practice. While guidelines referring to dual antiplatelet therapy (DAPT) after ACS with proceeding percutaneous coronary intervention (PCI) are uniform, there are doubts regarding DAPT after CABG, especially in setting of chronic coronary syndrome (CCS). Recommendations are mostly based on expert opinion and not on multiple randomized controlled trials (RCT) or meta-analyses. Resistance to aspirin (acetylsalicylic acid, ASA) or other antiplatelet drugs is known after CABG, and further RCTs are needed to assess the effect on clinical outcome as well as the role of DAPT after CABG.

Keywords: antiplatelet therapy, coronary artery bypass grafting (CABG), resistance to antiplatelet drugs, acute coronary syndrome (ACS), chronic coronary syndromes (CCS)

1. Introduction

An important and integral part of an optimal medicament therapy for patients with CAD in an acute as well as in a stable, chronic phase of the disease is antiplatelet therapy. The estimated number of patients requiring DAPT, consisting of a combination of ASA and an oral inhibitor of the platelet P2Y12 receptor for adenosine 5′-diphosphate (ADP), is considerable and has increased over time all around the world. Based on population estimates from 2015, in Europe 1.4–2.2 million patients per year may have an indication for DAPT after coronary intervention or myocardial infarction (MI), respectively [1]. There is, however, confusion about the optimal type and duration of DAPT in patients with established CAD, undergoing coronary revascularization or not. This derives from apparently conflicting results given in the available studies and limited evidence on various patient subsets [1]. Depending on the disease stage (ACS with PCI, CCS or coronary surgical revascularization), and comorbidity of each patient (e.g., atrial fibrillation, left ventricular thrombus, etc.), the strategy of antiplatelet/anticoagulant therapy is altered (combination of drugs, dosing, and duration of therapy). In patients with ACS treated with coronary stent implantation, DAPT is recommended for 12 months (preferring ticagrelor combined with ASA) [1]. In a patient with stable CAD treated with coronary stent implantation, DAPT consisting of clopidogrel in addition to aspirin is recommended for 6 months irrespective of the stent type (Class I, level of evidence A), and DAPT up to 12 months may be reasonable (Class IIb, level of evidence A) [1]. If treated with drug-coated balloon, DAPT (aspirin plus clopidogrel) should be considered for 6 months (Class IIa, level of evidence B) and prolonged up to 12 months in tolerant patients without bleeding complications [1]. As opposite, guidelines and especially clinical practice are not uniform and specific regarding patients who will undergo CABG. Latest guidelines regarding DAPT after CABG give general recommendation for duration and choice of antiplatelet therapy with relatively strong class of recommendation I or IIa/IIb[1]. Still, level of evidence in recommendations is mostly C or B[2] which points out that the foundation of recommendations is based on expert opinion and not on multiple RCTs or meta-analyses [1].

This chapter will give an overview of antiplatelet drugs, their mechanism of action, possible resistance to antiplatelet drugs, and clinical significance of resistance to antiplatelet drugs. Also, it will give an overview of literature regarding duration and choice of antiplatelet therapy after CABG in setting of ACS or CCS.

2. Antiplatelet therapy

2.1 Aspirin

Aspirin (acetylsalicylic acid, ASA) is classified among the nonsteroidal anti-inflammatory drugs (NSAIDs) and has analgesic, antipyretic, and antiplatelet properties. ASA achieves its effect primarily by interfering with the biosynthesis of cyclic prostanoids: thromboxane A2 (TXA2), prostacyclin, and other prostaglandins [2]. Low dose of ASA blocks the enzymatic effect of cyclooxygenase-1 (COX-1) on the transformation of arachidonic acid into prostaglandin G2 and then into prostaglandin H2 which is modified by specific synthases, producing prostaglandins and TXA2, an important mediator of the platelet aggregation response and in vasoconstriction [2–4]. One of the earliest placebo-controlled RCTs of ASA in patients with ACS consisted of 1266 men with unstable angina, and the combined primary end point of death and nonfatal MI at 12 weeks was reduced by 50% in patients receiving ASA rather than placebo [5]. The Second International Study of Infarct Survival (ISIS-2) study involving patients administered with daily 160-mg ASA started within the first day of MI and continued for 5 weeks and showed a significant risk reduction in total vascular mortality (23%) as well as a similar risk reduction of from all-cause mortality [6, 7]. Therapy with ASA has become regular for all patients suspected of having an ACS [7, 8].

[1] Class I, strong; Class IIa, moderate; Class IIb, weak; Class III, no benefit/harm.

[2] A, multiple RCTs/meta-analyses; B, single RCTs/large observational studies; C, expert opinion/small studies.

2.2 Clopidogrel

Clopidogrel is a second generation of thienopyridine antiplatelet agents and a P2RY12 inhibitor (purinergic receptor P2Y, G-protein coupled 12) which achieves its effect by irreversibly binding to the platelet P2RY12 receptor and blocking ADP-mediated platelet activation and aggregation [9]. It also inhibits collagen and thrombin-induced platelet aggregation which can be overcome by increased concentration of this agonist [10]. Clopidogrel versus aspirin in patients at risk of ischemic events (CAPRIE) trial demonstrated that long-term administration of clopidogrel to patients with atherosclerotic vascular disease is more effective than ASA in reducing the combined risk of ischemic stroke, MI, or vascular death, and the overall safety profile of clopidogrel is at least as good as that of medium-dose ASA [11]. The rate of reported gastrointestinal bleeding complication was significantly lower in the clopidogrel group than in the ASA group, and no difference in intracerebral hemorrhage, hemorrhagic death, thrombocytopenia, or neutropenia was noted between the two groups [7, 12]. Clopidogrel was then in 1997 approved by Food and Drug Administration (FDA) for use in secondary prevention of cardiovascular disease [7].

2.3 Ticagrelor

Ticagrelor is an orally administered direct-acting P2Y12-receptor antagonist [13, 14]. In vitro studies have demonstrated that ticagrelor binds reversibly and noncompetitively to the P2Y12 receptor at a site distinct from that of the endogenous agonist ADP [13]. In contrast, the thienopyridine compounds clopidogrel and prasugrel bind irreversibly to the P2Y12 receptor for the life of the platelet [15]. Ticagrelor was evaluated in patients with stable CAD in the Dose Confirmation Study Assessing Antiplatelet Effects of AZD6140 vs. Clopidogrel in Non–ST-Segment Elevation Myocardial Infarction (DISPERSE) trial [16]. In this randomized trial, patients with stable CAD who were taking ASA were administered either ticagrelor or clopidogrel, and after trial findings, the formulation of ticagrelor was changed, and the new corresponding doses of 90 mg and 180 mg twice a day were targeted in future studies [16, 17]. In the ONSET/OFFSET trial, the pharmacodynamic response of ticagrelor was assessed in patients with stable CAD, and significantly greater inhibition of platelet activation has been achieved in patients treated with ticagrelor plus ASA than with clopidogrel plus ASA [18].

2.4 Prasugrel

Prasugrel is an irreversible antagonist of the platelet ADP P2Y12 receptor and characterized by more potent antiplatelet effects, lower interindividual variability in platelet response, and faster onset of activity than clopidogrel [19]. The TRITON-TIMI 38 trial comparing prasugrel with clopidogrel in patients with moderate to high risk ACS (ST-elevation myocardial infarction, non-ST elevation myocardial infarction, and unstable angina) who underwent PCI demonstrated improved clinical outcomes with prasugrel as compared to clopidogrel [20]. A systematic review and recent meta-analysis suggest that prasugrel might have a better efficacy profile than ticagrelor in patients with ACS undergoing PCI, but this advantage was only seen in pooled observational studies and is likely to be affected by selection bias [21]. The latest trial comparing ticagrelor with prasugrel randomized 4018 patients which presented with ACS with or without ST-segment elevation (in whom invasive evaluation was planned), and the incidence of death, MI, or stroke was significantly lower among those who received prasugrel than among those who received ticagrelor, and the incidence of major bleeding was not significantly different between the two groups [22]. On the other hand, in the observational analysis of STEMI patients who underwent primary PCI, ticagrelor was associated with improved outcomes compared with clopidogrel and prasugrel [23].

3. Resistance to antiplatelet therapy and its clinical significance

The success of CABG depends mainly on the patency of the graft vessels; vein graft patency and disease have been shown to be closely related to long-term survival after CABG [24]. Vein graft disease consists of three different but related pathological processes: thrombosis, intimal hyperplasia, and atherosclerosis, where early thrombosis is a major cause of vein graft friction during the first month after CABG, while later on intimal hyperplasia is the leading cause of graft disease [25, 26]. Platelets participate in forming of blood clots, likewise they have an important role in graft thrombosis after CABG, and ASA is the primary antiplatelet drug that has been shown to improve vein graft patency within the first year after CABG [26–28]. Laboratory investigations showed that the expected inhibition of platelet function is not always achieved, which is called "aspirin nonresponse" or "aspirin resistance."

Speaking about nonresponse and resistance to aspirin, there are two terms in use. The first one is aspirin treatment failure which is defined as the occurrence of occlusive cardiovascular disease events despite the regular intake of aspirin in recommended doses [29]. Platelets are activated by many different pathways, and there are many factors that contribute to thrombotic event in addition to platelet aggregation. Occurrence of an ischemic event or treatment failure during single antiplatelet therapy is not synonymous with antiplatelet resistance. The second term is aspirin resistance or nonresponsiveness, and it is a laboratory phenomenon; therefore persistent presence of COX-1 activity after treatment with aspirin is an indicator of aspirin resistance [29]. Antiplatelet resistance to aspirin is only meaningful when it is highly associated with clinical outcomes. In a review article of antiplatelet treatment after CABG, a summary of benefit and failure of aspirin therapy is given [26]. It is emphasized that in the early period after CABG, increased risk of bypass thrombosis (among others, due to platelet activation and endothelial cell disruption of the graft) occurs simultaneously with increased prevalence of aspirin resistance [26, 30]. The underlying mechanisms of aspirin resistance are uncertain and largely hypothetical, i.e., increased platelet turnover, enhanced platelet reactivity, systemic inflammation, and drug–drug interaction are discussed [26, 31, 32]. It is also important to differentiate transient aspirin resistance after surgery from permanent aspirin nonresponse due to genetic polymorphisms [33] or comorbidities, such as hypercholesterolemia or diabetes [26, 34].

In clinical practice, patient nonadherence is the most common cause of aspirin nonresponse or treatment failure. Genetic variability and the number of single nucleotide polymorphism (SNPs) have been reported as the cause of aspirin resistance based on laboratory testing, but there is no evidence for strong relation between genetic variability and aspirin resistance [35]. Enteric-coated aspirin and delayed absorption may result in an insufficient antithrombotic effect, especially in the acute setting (pseudoresistance) [36]. Two studies (case–control, retrospective) have suggested that the use of proton pump inhibitors increases platelet aggregation and the risk of thrombotic events, but randomized trials are needed [37, 38]. Treatment failure attributable to other causes than genetic variability or lack of adherence is common. Functional and biochemical evaluation of platelet aspirin resistance in patients undergoing CABG suggested that aspirin resistance involves an impairment of both in vivo and in vitro inhibition of platelet functions and is probably due to a disturbed inhibition of platelet COX-1 by aspirin [39]. Aspirin resistance has been described in more than two-thirds of patients early after CABG [39, 40]. It has been shown that off-pump CABG (OPCABG) reduces platelet activation and turnover compared to on-pump CABG which may indicate that aspirin should be more effective after OPCABG [41], while other RCT showed no significant difference between off-pump and on-pump CABG in the rate of the 30-day composite outcome, but at 1 year of follow-up, patients in the off-pump group had worse composite outcomes and poorer graft patency [42]. In a group of patients with OPCABG, aspirin resistance was observed in nearly 30% on day 1 after OPCABG, but this is a transient phenomenon with only 4.5% of patients remaining so by postoperative day 10 [43]. The period of time passed after CABG is an important variable in measuring and analysis of the prevalence of aspirin resistance because results depend on it and vary from 10% up to >90% [26, 44, 45].

Regarding CABG, the number and size of trials investigating aspirin resistance with clinical endpoints are limited. A review of studies related to aspirin use after CABG suggested that clinical studies investigating the critical period early after CABG are necessary to correlate the results of reproducible assays with clinical outcomes that can possibly be improved by alterations in antiplatelet strategy [26]. The benefits and risks of ASA on thrombosis (BRAT) was the first prospective multicenter study with the objectives to determine the prevalence of aspirin responder or nonresponder status in patients undergoing CABG and to determine the clinical significance [46]. The 2-year follow-up period failed to show significant differences in thrombotic event rates (MI, unstable angina, cardiac death, or stroke) between aspirin responders and nonresponders [46]. In a setting of 225 patients undergoing elective OPCABG, aspirin resistance was defined by diagnostic findings on at least two of three separate assays (thromboelastography, whole blood aggregometry, and whole blood flow cytometry), and after multivariate logistic regression analysis, aspirin resistance on day 1 was retained as an independent predictor of vein graft thrombosis [47].

In the prospective randomized study to address the clinical impact of augmented antiplatelet therapy after elective CABG in patients with aggregometry-documented aspirin resistance, the addition of clopidogrel in patients found to be aspirin resistant after CABG did not reduce the incidence of adverse events, nor did it increase the number of recorded bleeding events [48]. A study on 60 patients who went to elective OPCABG and were divided into two groups to receive mono-antiplatelet treatment (MAPT) with ASA or DAPT with ASA and clopidogrel has shown that clopidogrel in addition to ASA reduces the incidence of OPCABG-related aspirin resistance, DAPT can be safely applied early after surgery, and there were no significant differences between two groups in postoperative bleeding [49]. A recent prospective, observational, bicentric cohort study indicated a high incidence of perioperative ASA nonresponse in patients following CABG, and no effect on the incidence of cardiovascular events was recorded in the 1-year follow-up [50]. Similar was concluded in a small low-risk cohort patients in which reduced ASA responsiveness as assessed with impedance aggregometry was not associated with increased incidence of major adverse cardiac and thromboembolic events and mortality after CABG surgery [51]. In a randomized trial on 68 patients, it was tested whether more frequent dosing improves ASA response following CABG surgery, and it was noted that twice-daily compared with once-daily dosing reduces ASA hyporesponsiveness after CABG surgery, but the efficacy of twice-daily ASA needs to be tested in a trial powered for clinical outcomes [52]. In comparison, meta-analyses of studies consisting of patients with cardiovascular disease (not only CABG patients) suggested that patients who were resistant to aspirin were at a greater risk of clinically important cardiovascular morbidity long term than patients who were sensitive to aspirin [53–55].

Concerning clopidogrel, patients with "high on-treatment platelet reactivity" (HPR) are divided into groups—nonresponsive, hyporesponsive, or resistant [56]. The term resistance or nonresponsiveness to an antiplatelet drug is used to describe a pharmacodynamics phenomenon where there is no clinically meaningful change in platelet function after treatment as compared with the baseline. In studies where light transmittance aggregometry was used, a change in maximal aggregation ≤10 percent from baseline, using ADP as the agonist, is defined as "resistance" [56]. In a systematic review of literature on clinical importance of ASA and clopidogrel resistance, almost all included studies have suggested a positive association between the risk of cardiovascular events and laboratory antiplatelet nonresponsiveness, and it was concluded that specific treatment recommendations are not established for patients who exhibit HPR during aspirin/clopidogrel therapy or who have poor platelet inhibition by clopidogrel [57]. A meta-analysis provided evidence that P2Y12 G52T/C34T polymorphism is related to a poor response of clopidogrel in patients; also a lack of association between T744C polymorphism and clopidogrel resistance was found [58]. Clopidogrel response in patients undergoing CABG remains unknown due to the fact that ASA is the drug of first choice after CABG, and clopidogrel administration (in addition to ASA) is recommended mainly in patients with ACS. However, previous reports indicate that the clopidogrel resistance rate in coronary stent patients varies between 5 and 56% [59]. Prospective, observational study on clopidogrel platelet reactivity in 859 patients who underwent OPCABG demonstrates that high residual platelet reactivity after clopidogrel administration is strongly associated with 1-year major adverse cardiovascular events (MACE)-free survival, and incidence of late MACEs was significantly higher in the HPR group than in the low platelet reactivity group, as such routine measurement of platelet reactivity and thorough monitoring of patients with HPR after OPCAB are suggested [60].

The latest review of literature on resistance to P2Y12 receptor antagonism in CAD showed that the prevalence of HPR is greater in patients treated with clopidogrel (approximately 30%) than in patients on the more novel antiplatelet agents prasugrel (3–15%) and ticagrelor (0–3%) [61]. Although meta-analyses show an effect of adjusting standard clopidogrel treatment based on platelet function testing, personalized therapy is not recommended because no large-scale RCT have shown any clinical benefit [61]. Nevertheless, it should be noticed that the performed RCTs were underpowered to show any clinical effect, and personalized therapy is recommended neither for patients on prasugrel nor those on ticagrelor due to low occurrence of HPR on these respective drugs [61]. The pharmacodynamic response of ticagrelor in clopidogrel nonresponders with stable CAD was assessed in an RCT: The response to ticagrelor in clopidogrel nonresponders and responders and effect of switching therapies (RESPOND) trial [62]. Inhibition of platelet function was significantly increased in clopidogrel nonresponders treated with ticagrelor compared with clopidogrel, and platelet aggregation decreased from 59 to 35% in patients who switched from clopidogrel to ticagrelor [62]. Despite the low platelet reactivity for both agents, comparisons have shown that ticagrelor is the most potent platelet inhibitor and has the lowest prevalence of HPR [63, 64]. Prasugrel resistance or variability in response is not clearly defined and depends on the in vitro system use, prasugrel resistance has been reported to occur in very few cases, and the mechanism of prasugrel resistance is still under investigation [65]. Despite small studies that have shown a few prasugrel-resistant patients due to low inhibition of platelet aggregation, the clinical significance of this phenomenon remains uncertain [65].

3.1 Platelet function tests for monitoring antiplatelet agent therapy

Platelet function testing is traditionally done to identify congenital and acquired platelet function defects. It is considered qualitative testing requiring interpretation in the context of patient condition. There exist multiple methods, each with its advantages and disadvantages.

Six major platelet function tests are most commonly used in the assessment of the prevalence of aspirin resistance in patients with stable CAD:

- Light transmission aggregometry (LTA) after stimulation arachidonic acid (AA)
- LTA after ADP stimulation
- Whole blood aggregometry
- PFA-100®
- VerifyNow Aspirin®
- Urinary 11-dehydro-thromboxane B2 concentrations that are measured [66]

4. CABG and antiplatelet therapy

CABG is an effective treatment for left main or multivessel ischemic heart disease, but long-term results are compromised by the development of saphenous vein graft (SVG) disease. ASA has always been a golden standard to prevent graft occlusion and adverse cardiac events after CABG [67]. DAPT was assessed in previous trials, but there is no clear evidence regarding its utility after CABG for preserving graft patency and reducing adverse cardiac events, especially in patients with stable ischemic heart disease (SIDH), recently referred as CCS. In the next subsections, it will be given an overview of available literature about efficacy of DAPT in preserving graft patency in setting of SIDH and CCS.

4.1 Antiplatelet therapy after CABG in setting of ACS

DAPT using ASA with either clopidogrel or ticagrelor is a standard of care for patients after ACS whether they were treated with PCI or medicament therapy only, preferring ticagrelor over clopidogrel [1, 68–71]. Latest guidelines recommend use of DAPT 1 year after CABG for patients with ACS [1, 71], although available evidence is limited to small RCTs and meta-analyses are substudies of larger RTCs. However, the choice between ASA and which P2Y12 inhibitor to use remains unclear in CABG. Synergistic antithrombotic effect of clopidogrel with ASA after ACS was evaluated in Unstable Angina to Prevent Recurrent Events (CURE) trial [72, 73]. Treatment with DAPT (ASA + clopidogrel) reduced the risk of the primary composite outcome—MI and recurrent ischemia, cerebrovascular event, and death from cardiovascular causes (MACCE), but the risk of major bleeding is increased among patients treated with clopidogrel [72]. The postoperative benefit with DAPT was analyzed in subgroup of CURE patients who underwent CABG and then were randomized to ASA and to ASA and clopidogrel. The benefits of DAPT with ASA and clopidogrel were consistent among groups undergoing CABG, PCI, or medical therapy, although the impact of DAPT among CABG patients did not reach significance for the primary composite outcome [73]. In a nationwide Danish cohort of real-life patients revascularized with CABG after MI, the benefit and efficacy of postoperative clopidogrel treatment in reducing risk of death or recurrent MI were confirmed [74]. The Platelet Inhibition and Patient Outcomes (PLATO) trial randomized patients with ACS to DAPT with either ASA plus ticagrelor 90 mg twice daily or ASA plus clopidogrel 75 mg once daily [75]. The composite primary end point of death from vascular causes, MI, or stroke was significantly reduced in the ticagrelor group, and ticagrelor was associated with a higher rate of major bleeding (no statistical difference in overall major bleeding). In a subgroup of patients who underwent CABG, effect on the primary outcome at 1 year was again consistent but did not reach significance. Cardiovascular mortality and all-cause mortality were significantly lower with ticagrelor, and there was no significant statistical benefit of ticagrelor related to MI and stroke [75]. DAPT with clopidogrel and ticagrelor in patients with non ST-elevation acute coronary syndrome (NSTE-ACS) was evaluated 3 months after off-pump CABG (only arterial grafts were used) in retrospective observational study, and there was no significant difference in overall survival or composite outcome of MACCE or major bleeding [76]. Prasugrel was compared with clopidogrel in patients with acute coronary syndrome RCT (TRITON-TIMI 38) where DAPT with ASA plus clopidogrel 75 mg daily or ASA plus prasugrel 10 mg daily was used [77]. Although major bleeding complications were significantly higher with prasugrel, the primary composite outcome of MACCE was significantly lower in prasugrel group, and all-cause mortality within 30 days in a subgroup of patients undergoing CABG was significantly reduced [77]. Meta-analysis of nine RCT that confirms benefit of DAPT among the subset of patients after ACS who had undergone CABG suggests that higher-intensity (prasugrel or ticagrelor) than lower-intensity (clopidogrel) DAPT is associated with an approximate 50% lower all-cause mortality in such patients, but data are primarily based on post-randomization subset from a single RCT [78]. Latest review on DAPT and CABG with focus on ACS supports the use of DAPT with ASA and ticagrelor for patients with ACS after CABG [79].

4.2 Antiplatelet therapy after CABG in setting of CCS

Stable ischemic heart disease (SIHD) refers to patients with known or suspected ischemic heart disease, including those with new-onset chest pain and those who have undergone PCI or CABG, and this term is used in 2014 ACC/AHA/AATS/PCNA/SCAI/STS Focused Update of the Guideline for the Diagnosis and Management of Patients With Stable Ischemic Heart Disease [80]. However, the disease is chronic, most often progressive and serious, even in clinically apparently silent periods. The new 2019 ESC Guidelines for the diagnosis and management of chronic coronary syndromes (CCS) emphasize that the dynamic nature of the CAD process results in various clinical presentations, which can be conveniently categorized as either ACS or CCS [81]. Latest guidelines note limited evidence on the role of DAPT after CABG in SIHD [1, 71]. 2016 ACC/AHA DAPT guideline update provides a class IIb recommendation for 12 months of DAPT to improve SVG patency [71]. The 2017 ESC focused update guideline suggests insufficient evidence to generally recommend DAPT postoperatively to reduce vein graft occlusion in stable patients who underwent CABG, unless concomitant or prior indication overrides [1]. Several studies have provided conflicting results on the effects of DAPT on the SVG patency. Graft patency was assessed with invasive coronary angiography or computerized tomography (CT). In Clopidogrel After Surgery for Coronary Artery disease (CASCADE) randomized trial, the combination of aspirin plus clopidogrel did not significantly reduce the process of SVG intimal hyperplasia (assessed with coronary angiography and intravascular ultrasound, IVUS) compared with ASA monotherapy [82]. Graft patency was not significantly improved in ROOBY trial [83] and a trial that randomized 100 patients after CABG [84]. In secondary analysis of CASCADE, the superiority of DAPT over ASA monotherapy in reducing the incidence of new occlusions within native coronary arteries after CABG was demonstrated [85]. Contradictorily, in Prevention of Coronary Artery Bypass Occlusion After Off-Pump Procedure (CRYSSA) trial, DAPT with ASA and clopidogrel was associated with significantly lower SVG occlusion rates than ASA monotherapy [86], and similar was shown in a previous RCT but with no significant differences in MACCE [87]. Observational studies in the cardiac surgery literature have suggested that clopidogrel may improve postoperative outcomes [88] and also demonstrated that the addition of clopidogrel to ASA was associated with a trend toward improved SVG patency 6 months after surgery [89], and it noted that postoperative clopidogrel was associated with less symptom recurrence and fewer adverse cardiac events [90]. Meta-analysis of DAPT with clopidogrel and ASA over monotherapy with ASA established that DAPT reduces the risk of SVG occlusion [91, 92] and was associated with a smaller incidence of early mortality but also linked with major bleeding episodes in the early postoperative period [92]. There is lack of studies that compare the effect of ticagrelor or prasugrel in addition to ASA on SVG patency. Effect of ticagrelor plus aspirin, ticagrelor alone, or aspirin alone on SVG patency 1 year after elective CABG was assessed in RCT and demonstrated that DAPT with ticagrelor and aspirin significantly improved graft patency, but there was no significant improvement with ticagrelor alone or aspirin alone, no statistically significant difference in event rates of MACCE, and no major bleeding in DAPT group [93]. And most recently, the Ticagrelor Compared with Aspirin for Prevention of Vascular Events in Patients Undergoing Coronary Artery Bypass Grafting (TiCAB) trial randomized patients in either ticagrelor twice daily or aspirin once daily group (study did not evaluate DAPT), and the primary outcome of MACE at 12 months did not differ significantly between two groups [94]. In latest meta-analyses data were also contradictory. One meta-analysis showed that DAPT appears to be associated with a reduction in graft occlusion and major adverse cardiac events in all-cause mortality, without significantly increasing major bleeding [95]. Improved graft patency with DAPT compared with aspirin was also shown in a meta-analysis of RCTs only [96]. Combined meta-analysis among patients undergoing CABG suggested association of DAPT with lover cardiovascular mortality in observational studies, but such findings were not replicated in RCTs [97].

4.3 Triple therapy (aspirin, P2Y12 inhibitor, and OAC) in patients after PCI or CABG

Addition of DAPT to oral anticoagulant (OAC) therapy increases bleeding complications for two- to threefolds [98, 99]. Therefore, patients who need triple therapy (comorbidity such as atrial fibrillation, thrombus in left ventricle, deep venous thrombosis, mechanical heart valve) are at high risk of bleeding. Assessing ischemic and bleeding risks using validated risk predictors (e.g., CHA_2DS_2-VASc[3], ABC[4], HAS-BLED[5]) with a focus on modifiable risk factors is one of the strategies to avoid bleeding complications. Triple therapy in patients undergoing PCI should last as short as possible (1 month if concerns about bleeding risks are prevailing and up

[3] CHA2DS2-VASc indicates congestive heart failure, hypertension, age ≥75 years (doubled), diabetes mellitus, prior stroke or transient ischemic attack or thromboembolism (doubled), vascular disease, age 65–74 years, and sex category.

[4] Age, biomarkers (GDF-15, cTnT-hs, hemoglobin), and clinical history (ABC).

[5] Hypertension, abnormal renal and liver function, stroke, bleeding, labile INR, elderly, drugs or alcohol (HAS-BLED).

to 6 months if concerns about ischemic risks are prevailing), and then dual therapy is to be considered (OAC and clopidogrel) up to 12 months [1]. Non-vitamin K oral anticoagulant (NOAC) should be considered instead of vitamin K antagonist (VKA). International normalized ratio (INR) is suggested to be in the lower part of the recommended target range, and time in therapeutic range should be maximized (i.e., >65–70%) when VKA is used [1, 71]. Using low dose (≤100 mg) of ASA is recommended and also routine use of proton pump inhibitors (PPIs) [1, 71]. Clopidogrel is the P2Y12 inhibitor of choice in such regimen of therapy; the use of prasugrel and ticagrelor should be avoided [1]. In a study of 377 patients who underwent drug-eluting stent implantation and had an indication for oral anticoagulation, prasugrel was evaluated as alternative to clopidogrel, and results showed an increased risk of bleeding in patients needing triple therapy [100]. Recent meta-analysis demonstrated that the use of ticagrelor as part of dual or triple therapy is associated with significantly higher rates of clinically relevant hemorrhagic complications than clopidogrel [101]. Latest review article on this subject points out already known stronger antiplatelet effect of ticagrelor and prasugrel, yet they are not used because of the increased risk, whether real or perceived, which has not been confirmed with large RCT in patients with ACS and atrial fibrillation [102]. In patients eligible for CABG surgery, DAPT should be avoided on the top of OAC and is not suggested in which antiplatelet agent in addition to OAC should be used [1].

5. Conclusion

- There is no strong evidence based on RCTs or meta-analysis regarding duration and choice of antiplatelet agents after CABG, especially in setting of stable CAD.

- The 2017 ESC focused update guideline suggests insufficient evidence to generally recommend DAPT postoperatively to reduce graft occlusion in stable patients who underwent CABG, unless concomitant or prior indication overrides. In setting of ACS, combination of ASA with P2Y12 inhibitor is recommended up to 12 months after CABG, but the choice between ASA and which P2Y12 inhibitor to use is not clearly defined. In patients perceived at high ischemic risk with prior MI and CABG who have tolerated DAPT without bleeding complications, treatment with DAPT for longer than 12 months and up to 36 months may be considered [1].

- There is no clear evidence of aspirin resistance in CABG patients and effect on their clinical outcome. Also, there is no uniform data regarding addition of clopidogrel to ASA in reducing the incidence of CABG-related aspirin resistance.

- Available data suggests that the incidence of late MACEs was higher in the HPR group after clopidogrel administration post CABG, and also higher prevalence of HPR was shown in CAD patients treated with clopidogrel than patients treated with ticagrelor or prasugrel. Positive effect of adjusting standard clopidogrel treatment based on platelet function testing was shown; however, personalized therapy is not recommended because no large RCT demonstrated any clinical benefit.

- Ticagrelor and prasugrel have a low occurrence of HPR, and platelet function testing is not recommended; in addition there are no large RCT studies available on this subject.

- Resistance to antiplatelet drugs and its impact to the clinical outcomes (bypass patency, major adverse cardiovascular events such as MI, PCI, re-do CABG, and cardiac mortality) of patients requires further investigation with larger studies.

- It is reasonable to assume (and meta-analyses of studies consisting of patients with cardiovascular disease suggest) that patients who are resistant to ASA have a greater risk of clinically important cardiovascular morbidity long term than ASA-sensitive patients.

- Further studies are needed in order to define the role of more aggressive antiplatelet therapy post CABG on graft patency and clinical outcome.

- Besides optimal antiplatelet therapy, other variables such as surgeon experience and skill, stage and severity of CAD, long-lasting postoperative control of cardiovascular risk factors, the degree of reduction of systolic function of left ventricle before CABG, and other associated comorbidity (e.g., diabetes, chronic renal failure, etc.) have to be taken into consideration when interpreting MACCE and CABG patient outcomes.

Author details

Ivana Sopek Merkas[1*], Nenad Lakusic[1,2,3], Krunoslav Fuckar[1,2], Dusko Cerovec[1,2] and Kristina Maric Besic[4,5]

1 Special Hospital for Medical Rehabilitation Krapinske Toplice, Krapinske Toplice, Croatia

2 Faculty of Medicine Osijek, Josip Juraj Strossmayer University of Osijek, Osijek, Croatia

3 Faculty of Dental Medicine and Health Osijek, Josip Juraj Strossmayer University of Osijek, Osijek, Croatia

4 University Hospital Centre Zagreb, Zagreb, Croatia

5 Faculty of Medicine Zagreb, University of Zagreb, Zagreb, Croatia

*Address all correspondence to: ivana.sopek92@gmail.com

References

[1] Valgimigli M, Bueno H, Byrne RA, et al. 2017 ESC focused update on dual antiplatelet therapy in coronary artery disease developed in collaboration with EACTS: the Task Force for dual antiplatelet therapy in coronary artery disease of the European Society of Cardiology (ESC) and of the European Association for Cardio-Thoracic Surgery (EACTS). European Heart Journal. 2018;**39**:213-254. DOI: 10.1093/eurheartj/ehx419

[2] Awtry EH, Loscalzo J. Aspirin. Circulation. 2000;**101**:1206-1218

[3] Vane JR. Inhibition of prostaglandin synthesis as a mechanism of action for aspirin-like drugs. Nature New Biology. 1971;**231**:232-235. DOI: 10.1038/newbio231232a0

[4] Burch JW, Stanford N, Majerus PW. Inhibition of platelet prostaglandin synthetase by oral aspirin. Journal of Clinical Investigation. 1978;**61**:314-319. DOI: 10.1172/JCI108941

[5] Lewis HD, Davis JW, Archibald DG, et al. Protective effects of aspirin against acute myocardial infarction and death in men with unstable angina: Results of a veterans administration cooperative study. New England Journal of Medicine. 1983;**309**:396-403. DOI: 10.1056/NEJM198308183090703

[6] ISIS-2 (Second International Study of Infarct Survival) Collaborative Group. Randomized trial of intravenous streptokinase, oral aspirin, both, or neither among 17 187 cases of suspected acute myocardial infarction: ISIS-2. The Lancet. 1988;**332**:349-360. DOI: 10.1016/S0140-6736(88)92833-4

[7] Jneid H, Batt DL, Corti R, et al. Aspirin and clopidogrel in acute coronary syndromes; therapeutic insights from the CURE study. Archives of Internal Medicine. 2003;**163**(10):1145-1153. DOI: 10.1001/archinte.163.10.1145

[8] Hennekens CH, Dyken ML, Fuster V, et al. Aspirin as a therapeutic agent in cardiovascular disease: A statement for healthcare professionals from the American Heart Association. Circulation. 1997, 2753;**96**:2751. DOI: 0.1161/01.CIR.96.8.2751

[9] Herbert JM, Frehel D, Kieffer G, et al. Clopidogrel, a novel antiplatelet and antithrombotic agent. Cardiovascular Drug Reviews. 1993;**11**:180-198. DOI: 10.1111/j.1527-3466.1993.tb00275.x

[10] Shuvan R. Clopidogrel resistance: The way forward. Indian Heart Journal. 2014;**66**:530-534. DOI: 10.1016/j.ihj.2014.08.012

[11] Gent M, CAPRIE Steering Committee. A randomized, blinded, trial of clopidogrel versus aspirin in patients at risk of ischemic events (CAPRIE). The Lancet. 1996;**348**:1329-1339. DOI: 10.1016/S0140-6736(96)09457-3

[12] Creager MA. Results of the CAPRIE trial: Efficacy and safety of clopidogrel: Clopidogrel versus aspirin in patients at risk of ischemic events. Vascular Medicine. 1998:3257-3260. DOI: 10.1177/1358836X9800300314

[13] van Giezen JJ, Nilsson L, Berntsson P, et al. Ticagrelor binds to human P2Y(12) independently from ADP but antagonizes ADP-induced receptor signaling and platelet aggregation. Journal of Thrombosis and Haemostasis. 2009;**7**:1556-1565. DOI: 10.1111/j.1538-7836.2009.03527.x

[14] Husted S, van Giezen JJ. Ticagrelor: The first reversibly binding oral P2Y12 receptor antagonist. Cardiovascular

Therapeutics. 2009;**27**:259-274. DOI: 10.1111/j.1755-5922.2009.00096.x

[15] van Giezen JJ, Berntsson P, Zachrisson H, et al. Comparison of ticagrelor and thienopyridine P2Y(12) binding characteristics and antithrombotic and bleeding effects in rat and dog models of thrombosis/hemostasis. Thrombosis Research. 2009;**124**:565-571. DOI: 10.1016/j.thromres.2009.06.029

[16] Husted S, Emanuelsson H, Heptinstall S, et al. Pharmacodynamics, pharmacokinetics, and safety of the oral reversible P2Y12 antagonist AZD6140 with aspirin in patients with atherosclerosis: A double-blind comparison to clopidogrel with aspirin. European Heart Journal. 2006;**27**:1038-1047. DOI: 10.1093/eurheartj/ehi754

[17] Dobesh PP, Oestreich JH. Ticagrelor: Pharmacokineticks,pharmacodynamics, clinical efficacy and safety. Pharmacotherapy. 2014;**34**:1077-1090. DOI: 10.1002/phar.1477

[18] Gurbel PA, Bliden KP, Butler K, et al. Randomized double-blind assessment of the ONSET and OFFSET of the antiplatelet effects of ticagrelor versus clopidogrel in patients with stable coronary artery disease: The ONSET/OFFSET study. Circulation. 2009;**120**:2577-2585. DOI: 10.1161/CIRCULATIONAHA.109.912550

[19] Mousa SA, Jeske PW, Fareed J. Antiplatelet therapy prasugrel: A novel platelet ADP P2Y12 receptor antagonist. Clinical and Applied Thrombosis/Hemostasis. 2010;**16**:170-176. DOI: 10.1177/1076029609355589

[20] Montalescot G, Wiviott SD, Braunwald E, et al. Prasugrel compared with clopidogrel in patients undergoing percutaneous coronary intervention for ST-elevation myocardial infarction TRITON-TIMI 38: Double-blind, randomized controlled trial. Lancet. 2009;**373**(9665):723-731

[21] Khan MS, Memon MM, Usman MS, et al. Prasugrel vs. ticagrelor for acute coronary syndrome patients undergoing percutaneous coronary intervention: A systematic review and meta-analysis. American Journal of Cardiovascular Drugs. 2019;**19**:465-476. DOI: 10.1007/s40256-019-00337-5

[22] Schupke S, Neumann FJ, Menichelli M, et al. Ticagrelor or prasugrel in patients with acute coronary syndromes. New England Journal of Medicine. 2019;**381**:1524-1534. DOI: 10.1056/NEJMoa1908973

[23] Welsh RC, Sidhu RS, Cairns JA, et al. Outcomes among clopidogrel, prasugrel, and ticagrelor in ST-elevation myocardial infarction patients who underwent primary percutaneous coronary intervention: From the TOTAL trial. Canadian Journal of Cardiology. 2019;**35**:1377-1385. DOI: 10.1016/j.cjca.2019.04.026

[24] Fitzgibbon GM, Kafka HP, Leach AJ, et al. Coronary bypass graft fate and patient outcome: Angiographic follow-up of 5,065 grafts related to survival and reoperation in 1,388 patients during 25 years. Journal of American College of Cardiology. 1996;**28**:616-626. DOI: 10.1016/0735-1097(96)00206-9

[25] Motwani JG, Topol EJ. Aortocoronary saphenous vein graft disease: Pathogenesis, predisposition and prevention. Circulation. 1998;**97**:916-931. DOI: 10.1161/01.cir.97.9.916

[26] Zimmermann N, Gams E, Hohlfeld T. Aspirin in coronary artery bypass surgery: New aspects of and alternatives for an old antithrombotic agent. European Journal of Cardio-Thoracic Surgery. 2008;**34**:93-108. DOI: 10.1016/j.ejcts.2008.03.023

[27] Goldman S, Copeland J, Moritz T, et al. Improvement in early saphenous vein graft patency after coronary artery bypass surgery with antiplatelet therapy: Results of a veterans administration cooperative study. Circulation. 1988;77:1324-1332. DOI: 10.1161/01.CIR.77.6.1324

[28] Goldman S, Copeland J, Moritz T, et al. Saphenous vein graft patency 1 year after coronary artery bypass surgery and effects of antiplatelet therapy. Results of a veterans administration cooperative study. Circulation. 1989;**80**:1190-1197. DOI: 10.1161/01.CIR.80.5.1190

[29] Michelson AD, Cattaneo M, Eikelboom JW, et al. Aspirin resistance: Position paper of the working group on aspirin resistance. Journal of Thrombosis and Haemostasis. 2005;**3**:1309. DOI: 10.1111/j.1538-7836.2005.01351.x

[30] Guthikonda S, Lev EI, Patel R, et al. Reticulated platelets and uninhibited COX-1 and COX-2 decrease the antiplatelet effects of aspirin. Journal of Thrombosis and Haemostasis. 2007;**5**:490-496. DOI: 10.1111/j.1538-7836.2007.02387.x

[31] Raja SG, Berg GA. Impact of off-pump coronary artery bypass surgery on systemic inflammation: Current best available evidence. Journal of Cardiac Surgery. 2007;**22**:445-455. DOI: 10.1111/j.1540-8191.2007.00447.x

[32] Catella-Lawson F, Reilly MP, Kapoor SC, et al. Cyclooxygenase inhibitors and the antiplatelet effects of aspirin. New England Journal of Medicine. 2001;**345**:1809-1817. DOI: 10.1056/NEJMoa003199

[33] Marin F, Roldan V, Gonzalez-Conejero R, et al. The pharmacogenetics of antiplatelet drugs. Current Opinion in Investigational Drugs. 2007;**8**:213-218

[34] Davi G, Gresele P, Violi F, et al. Diabetes mellitus, hypercholesterolemia, and hypertension but not vascular disease per se are associated with persistent platelet activation in vivo. Evidence derived from the study of peripheral arterial disease. Circulation. 1997;**96**:69-75. DOI: 10.1161/01.CIR.96.1.69

[35] Voora D, Horton J, Shah SH, et al. Polymorphisms associated with in vitro aspirin resistance are not associated with clinical outcomes in patients with coronary artery disease who report regular aspirin use. American Heart Journal. 2011;**162**:166-172. DOI: 10.1016/j.ahj.2011.03.026

[36] Grosser T, Fries S, Lawson JA, et al. Drug resistance and pseudoresistance: An unintended consequence of enteric coating aspirin. Circulation. 2013;**127**:377-385. DOI: 10.1161/CIRCULATIONAHA.112.117283

[37] Würtz M, Gove EL, Kristensen SD, Hvas AM. The antiplatelet effect of aspirin is reduced by proton pump inhibitors in patients with coronary artery disease. Heart. 2010;**96**:368-371. DOI: 10.1136/hrt.2009.181107

[38] Charlot M, Grove EL, Hansen PR, et al. Proton pump inhibitor use and risk of adverse cardiovascular events in aspirin treated patients with first time myocardial infarction: Nationwide propensity score matched study. BMJ. 2011;**342**:d2690. DOI: 10.1136/bmj.d2690

[39] Zimmermann N, Wenk A, Kim U, et al. Functional and biochemical evaluation of platelet aspirin resistance after coronary artery bypass surgery. Circulation. 2003;**108**:542-547. DOI: 10.1161/01.CIR.0000081770.51929.5A

[40] Poston RS, Gu J, White C, et al. Perioperative management of aspirin resistance after off-pump

coronary artery bypass grafting: Possible role for aprotinin. Transfusion. 2008;**48**:39S-46S. DOI: 10.1111/j.1537-2995.2007.01575.x

[41] Ballotta A, Saleh HZ, El Baghdady HW, et al. Comparison of early platelet activation in patients undergoing on-pump versus off-pump coronary artery bypass surgery. Journal of Thoracic and Cardiovascular Surgery. 2007;**134**:132-138. DOI: 10.1016/j.jtcvs.2007.01.055

[42] Shroyer AL, Grover FL, Hattler B, et al. Veterans Affairs Randomized On/Off Bypass (Rooby) Study Group. On-pump versus off-pump coronary artery bypass surgery. The New England Journal of Medicine. 2009;**361**:1827-1837. DOI: 10.1056/NEJMoa0902905

[43] Wang Z, Gao F, Men J, et al. Aspirin resistance in off-pump coronary artery bypass grafting. European Journal of Cardio-Thoracic Surgery. 2012;**41**:108-112. DOI: 10.1016/j.ejcts.2011.04.021

[44] Golanski J, Chlopicki S, Golanski R, et al. Resistance to aspirin in patients after coronary artery bypass grafting is transient: Impact on the monitoring of aspirin antiplatelet therapy. Therapeutic Drug Monitoring. 2005;**27**:484-490. DOI: 10.1097/01.ftd.0000158084.84071.41

[45] Zimmermann N, Kurt M, Winter J, et al. Detection and duration of aspirin resistance after coronary artery bypass grafting. Journal of Thoracic and Cardiovascular Surgery. 2008;**135**:947-948. DOI: 10.1016/j.jtcvs.2007.11.033

[46] Buchanan M, Schwartz L, Bourassa M, et al. BRAT investigators. Results of the BRAT study: A pilot study investigating the possible significance of ASA non responsiveness on the benefits and risks of ASA on thrombosis in patients undergoing coronary artery bypass surgery. Canadian Journal of Cardiology. 2000;**16**:1385-1390

[47] Poston RS, Gu J, Brown JM, Gammie JS, et al. Endothelial injury and acquired aspirin resistance as promoters of regional thrombin formation and early vein graft failure after coronary artery bypass grafting. Journal of Thoracic and Cardiovascular Surgery. 2006;**131**:122-130. DOI: 10.1016/j.jtcvs.2005.08.058

[48] Gasparovic H, Petricevic M, Kopjar T, et al. Impact of dual antiplatelet therapy on outcomes among aspirin-resistant patients following coronary artery bypass grafting. American Journal of Cardiology. 2014;**113**:1660-1667. DOI: 10.1016/j.amjcard.2014.02.024

[49] Wang X, Gong X, Zhu T, et al. Clopidogrel improves aspirin response after off-pump coronary artery bypass surgery. The Journal of Biomedical Research. 2014;**28**:108-113. DOI: 10.7555/JBR.28.20120139

[50] Wand S, Adam HE, Wetz JA, et al. The prevalence and clinical relevance of ASA nonresponse after cardiac surgery: A prospective bicentric study. Clinical and Applied Thrombosis/Hemostasis. 2018;**24**:179-185. DOI: 10.1177/1076029617693939

[51] Bolliger D, Filipovic M, Matt P, et al. Reduced aspirin responsiveness as assessed by impedance aggregometry is not associated with adverse outcome after cardiac surgery in a small low-risk cohort. Platelets. 2016;**27**:254-261. DOI: 10.3109/09537104.2015.1083969

[52] Paikin JS, Hirsh J, Ginsberg JS, et al. Once versus twice daily aspirin after coronary bypass surgery: A randomized trial. Journal of Thrombosis and Haemostasis. 2017;**15**:889-896. DOI: 10.1111/jth.13667

[53] Snoep JD, Hovens MM, Eikenboom JC, et al. Association of laboratory-defined aspirin resistance with a higher risk of recurrent

cardiovascular events: A systematic review and meta-analysis. Archives of Internal Medicine. 2007;**167**:1593-1599. DOI: 10.1001/archinte.167.15.1593

[54] Krasopoulos G, Brister SJ, Beattie WS, et al. Aspirin "resistance" and risk of cardiovascular morbidity: Systematic review and meta-analysis. BMJ. 2008;**336**:195-198. DOI: 10.1136/bmj.39430.529549.BE

[55] Sofi F, Marcucci R, Gori AM, et al. Residual platelet reactivity on aspirin therapy and recurrent cardiovascular events--a meta-analysis. International Journal of Cardiology. 2008;**128**:166-171. DOI: 10.1016/j.ijcard.2007.12.010

[56] Tantry US, Bliden KP, Gurbel PA. Resistance to antiplatelet drugs: Current status and future research. Expert Opinion Pharmacotherapy. 2005;**6**:2027-2045. DOI: 10.1517/14656566.6.12.2027

[57] Feher G, Feher A, Pusch G, et al. Clinical importance of aspirin and clopidogrel resistance. World Journal of Cardiology. 2010;**2**:171-186. DOI: 10.4330/wjc.v2.i7.171

[58] Cui G, Zhang C, Zou J, et al. P2Y12 receptor gene polymorphism and the risk of resistance to clopidogrel: A meta-analysis and review of the literature. Advances in Clinical and Experimental Medicine. 2017;**26**:343-349. DOI: 10.17219/acem/63745

[59] Serebruany VL, Steinhubl SR, Berger PB, et al. Variability in platelet responsiveness to clopidogrel among 544 individual. Journal of the American College of Cardiology. 2005;**45**:246-251. DOI: 10.1016/j.jacc.2004.09.067

[60] Youn YN, Yi G, Lee S, et al. Posttreatment platelet reactivity on clopidogrel is associated with the risk of adverse events after off-pump coronary artery bypass. American Heart Journal. 2014;**167**:818-825. DOI: 10.1016/j.ahj.2014.01.016

[61] Warlo EMK, Arnesen H, Seljeflot I. A brief review on resistance to P2Y12 receptor antagonism in coronary artery disease. Thrombosis Journal. 2019;**17**:11. DOI: 10.1186/s12959-019-0197-5

[62] Gurbel PA, Bliden KP, Butler K, et al. Response to ticagrelor in clopidogrel nonresponders and responders and effect of switching therapies: The RESPOND study. Circulation. 2010;**121**:1188-1199. DOI: 10.1161/CIRCULATIONAHA.109.919456

[63] Lhermusier T, Lipinski MJ, Tantry US, et al. Meta-analysis of direct and indirect comparison of ticagrelor and prasugrel effects on platelet reactivity. The American Journal of Cardiology. 2015;**115**:716-723. DOI: 10.1016/j.amjcard.2014.12.029

[64] Lemesle G, Schurtz G, Bauters C, et al. High on-treatment platelet reactivity with ticagrelor versus prasugrel: A systematic review and meta-analysis. Journal of Thrombosis and Haemostasis. 2015;**13**:931-942. DOI: 10.1111/jth.12907

[65] Sardella G, Calcagno S, Mancone M, et al. Comparison of therapy with ticagrelor, prasugrel or high clopidogrel dose in PCI patients with high on treatment platelet reactivity and genotype variation. TRIPLETE RESET trial. International Journal of Cardiology. 2015;**194**:60-62. DOI: 10.1016/j.ijcard.2015.05.085

[66] Lordkipanidzé M, Pharand C, Schampaert E, et al. A comparison of six major platelet function tests to determine the prevalence of aspirin resistance in patients with stable coronary artery disease. European Heart Journal. 2007;**28**:1702-1708. DOI: 10.1093/eurheartj/ehm226

[67] Kulik A, Ruel M, Jneid H, et al. Secondary prevention after coronary

bypass graft surgery: A scientific statement from the American Heart Association. Circulation. 2015;**131**:927-964. DOI: 10.1161/CIR.0000000000000182

[68] Mehta SR, Bainey KR, Cantor WJ, et al. 2018 Canadian Cardiovascular Society/Canadian Association of Interventional Cardiology focused update of the guidelines for the use of antiplatelet therapy. Canadian Journal of Cardiology. 2018;**34**:214-233. DOI: 10.1016/j.cjca.2017.12.012

[69] Amsterdam ES, Wenger NK, Brindis RG, et al. 2014 AHA/ACC guideline for the management of patients with non–ST-elevation acute coronary syndromes: A report of the American College of Cardiology/American Heart Association Task Force on Practice Guidelines. Journal of the American College of Cardiology. 2014;**64**:e139-e228. DOI: 10.1016/j.jacc.2014.09.017

[70] Roffi M, Patrono C, Collet JP, et al. 2015 ESC guidelines for the management of acute coronary syndromes in patients presenting without persistent ST-segment elevation: The Task Force for the management of acute coronary syndromes in patients presenting without persistent ST-segment elevation of the European Society of Cardiology (ESC). European Heart Journal. 2016;**37**:267-315. DOI: 10.1093/eurheartj/ehv320

[71] Levine GN, Bates ER, et al. 2016 ACC/AHA Guideline focused update on duration of dual antiplatelet therapy in patients with coronary artery disease: a report of the American College of Cardiology/American Heart Association; Task Force on Clinical Practice Guidelines. Journal of the American College of Cardiology. 2016;**68**:108-115. DOI: 10.1016/j.jacc.2016.03.513

[72] Yusuf S, Zhao F, Mehta SR, et al. Effects of clopidogrel in addition to aspirin in patients with acute coronary syndromes without ST-segment elevation. New England Journal of Medicine. 2001;**345**:494-502. DOI: 10.1056/NEJMoa010746

[73] Fox KA, Mehta SR, Peters R, et al. Benefits and risks of the combination of clopidogrel and aspirin in patients undergoing surgical revascularization for non–ST-elevation acute coronary syndrome: The Clopidogrel in unstable angina to prevent recurrent ischemic events (CURE) trial. Circulation. 2004;**110**:1202-1208. DOI: 10.1161/01.CIR.0000140675.85342.1B

[74] Sørensen R, Abildstrøm SZ, Hansen PR, et al. Efficacy of post-operative clopidogrel treatment in patients revascularized with coronary artery bypass grafting after myocardial infarction. Journal of the American College of Cardiology. 2011;**57**:1202-1209. DOI: 10.1016/j.jacc.2010.09.06

[75] Wallentin I, Becker RC, Budaj A, et al. Ticagrelor versus clopidogrel in patients with acute coronary syndromes. New England Journal of Medicine. 2009;**361**:1045-1057. DOI: 10.1056/NEJMoa0904327

[76] Chang HW, Kim HJ, Yoo JS, et al. Clopidogrel versus ticagrelor for secondary prevention after coronary artery bypass grafting. Journal of Clinical Medicine. 2019;**8**:104. DOI: 10.3390/jcm8010104

[77] Wiviott S, Braunwald E, McCabe CH, et al. Prasugrel versus clopidogrel in patients with acute coronary syndromes. New England Journal of Medicine. 2007;**357**:2001-2015. DOI: 10.1056/NEJMoa0706482

[78] Verma S, Goodman SG, Mehta SR, et al. Should dual antiplatelet therapy be used in patients following coronary artery bypass surgery? A meta-analysis of randomized controlled trials. BMC

Surgery. 2015;**15**:112. DOI: 10.1186/s12893-015-0096-z

[79] Gupta S, Belley-Cote EP, Agahi P, et al. Antiplatelet therapy and coronary artery bypass grafting: Analysis of current evidence with a focus on acute coronary syndorme. Canadian Journal of Cardiology. 2019;**35**:1030-1038. DOI: 10.1016/j.cjca.2019.06.003

[80] Fihn SD, James C, Blankenship JC, et al. 2014 ACC/AHA/AATS/PCNA/SCAI/STS focused update of the guideline for the diagnosis and management of patients with stable ischemic heart disease. Journal of the American College of Cardiology. 2014;**130**:1749-1767. DOI: 10.1161/CIR.0000000000000095

[81] Knuuti J, Wijns W, Saraste A, et al. 2019 ESC guidelines for the diagnosis and management of chronic coronary syndromes. European Heart Journal. 2019;pii:ehz425. DOI: 10.1093/eurheartj/ehz425. Available from: https://academic.oup.com/eurheartj/advance-article/doi/10.1093/eurheartj/ehz425/5556137

[82] Kulik A, Le May RM, Voisine P, et al. Aspirin plus clopidogrel after surgery for coronary artery disease (CASCADE) trial. Circulation. 2010;**122**:2680-2687. DOI: 10.1161/CIRCULATIONAHA.110.978007

[83] Ebrahimi R, Bakeen FG, Uberoi A. Effect of clopidogrel use post coronary artery bypass surgery on graft patency. The Annals of Thoracic Surgery. 2014;**97**:15-21. DOI: 10.1016/j.athoracsur.2013.08.058

[84] Sun JC, Teoh KH, Lamy A, et al. Randomized trial of aspirin and clopidogrel versus aspirin alone for the prevention of coronary artery bypass graft occlusion: The preoperative aspirin and postoperative antiplatelets in coronary artery bypass grafting study. American Heart Journal. 2010;**160**:1178-1184. DOI: 10.1016/j.ahj.2010.07.035

[85] Une D, Al-Atassi T, Kulik A, et al. Impact of clopidogrel plus aspirin versus aspirin alone on the progression of native coronary artery disease after bypass surgery analysis from the aspirin plus clopidogrel after surgery for coronary artery disease (CASCADE) randomized trial. Circulation. 2014;**130**:S12-S18. DOI: 10.1161/CIRCULATIONAHA.113.008227

[86] Mannacio VA, Di Tommaso L, Antignan A, et al. Aspirin plus clopidogrel for optimal platelet inhibition following off-pump coronary artery bypass surgery: Result from the CRYSSA (prevention of coronary artery bypass occlusion after off pump procedures) randomized study. Heart. 2012;**98**:1710-1715. DOI: 10.1136/heartjnl-2012-302449

[87] Gao G, Zheng Z, Lu B, et al. Aspirin plus clopidogrel therapy increases early venous graft patency after coronary artery bypass surgery. Journal of the American College of Cardiology. 2010;**56**:1639-1643. DOI: 10.1016/j.jacc.2010.03.104

[88] Kim DH, Daskalakis C, Silvestry SC, et al. Aspirin and clopidogrel use in the early postoperative period following on-pump and off-pump coronary artery bypass grafting. The Journal of Thoracic and Cardiovascular Surgery. 2009;**138**:1377-1384. DOI: 10.1016/j.jtcvs.2009.07.027

[89] Ibrahim K, Tjomsland O, Halvorsen D, et al. Effect of clopidogrel on midterm graft patency following off-pump coronary revascularization surgery. The Heart Surgery Forum. 2006;**9**:E581-E856. DOI: 10.1532/HSF98.20061034

[90] Gurbuz AT, Zia AA, Vuran AC, et al. Postoperative clopidogrel improves mid-term outcome after off-pump

coronary artery bypass graft surgery: A prospective study. European Journal of Cardio-Thoracic Surgery. 2006;**29**:190-195. DOI: 10.1016/j.ejcts.2005.11.033

[91] Nocerino AG, Achenbach S, Taylor AJ. Meta-analysis of effect of single versus dual antiplatelet therapy on early patency of bypass conduits after coronary artery bypass grafting. American Journal of Cardiology. 2013;**112**:1576-1579. DOI: 10.1016/j.amjcard.2013.07.017

[92] Deo SV, Dunnlay SM, Shah IK, et al. Dual anti-platelet therapy after coronary artery bypass grafting: Is there any benefit? A systematic review and meta-analysis. Journal of Cardiac Surgery. 2013;**28**:109-116. DOI: 10.1111/jocs.12074

[93] Zhao Q, Zhu Y, Xu Z, et al. Effect of ticagrelor plus aspirin, ticagrelor alone or aspirin alone on saphenous vein graft patency 1 year after coronary artery bypass grafting. JAMA. 2018;**319**:1677-1686. DOI: 10.1001/jama.2018.3197

[94] Schunkert H, Boening H, von Scheidt M, et al. Randomized trial of ticagrelor vs. aspirin in patients after coronary artery bypass grafting: The TiCAB trial. European Heart Journal. 2019;**40**:2432-2440. DOI: 10.1093/eurheartj/ehz185

[95] Agrawal N, Mahmoud AN, Patel KN, et al. Meta-analysis of aspirin versus dual antiplatelet therapy following coronary artery bypass grafting. American Journal of Cardiology. 2018;**121**:32-40. DOI: 10.1016/j.amjcard.2017.09.022

[96] Chakos A, Jbara D, Singh K, et al. Network meta-analysis of antiplatelet therapy following coronary artery bypass grafting (CABG): None versus one versus two antiplatelet agents. Anals of Cardiothoracic Surgery. 2018;7:577-585. DOI: 10.21037/acs.2018.09.02

[97] Cardoso R, Knijnik L, Whelton SP, et al. Dual versus single antiplatelet therapy after coronary artery bypass graft surgery: An updated meta-analysis. International Journal of Cardiology. 2018;**269**:80-88. DOI: 10.1016.j.ijcard.2018.07.083

[98] Sorensen R, Hansen ML, Abildstrom SZ, et al. Risk of bleeding in patients with acute myocardial infarction treated with different combinations of aspirin, clopidogrel and vitamin K antagonist in Denmark: A retrospective analysis of nationwide registry data. Lancet. 2009;**374**:1967-1974. DOI: 10.1016/S0140-6736(09)61751-7

[99] Hansen ML, Sorensen R, Clausen MT, et al. Risk of bleeding with single, dual or triple therapy with warfarin, aspirin and clopidogrel in patients with atrial fibrillation. Archives of Internal Medicine. 2010;**170**:1433-1441. DOI: 10.1001/archinternmed.2010.271

[100] Sarafoff N, Martisching A, Wealer J, et al. Triple therapy with aspirin, prasugrel and vitamin K antagonists in patients with drug-eluting stent implantation and an indication for oral anticoagulation. Journal of the American College of Cardiology. 2013;**61**:2016-2066. DOI: 10.1016/j.jacc.2013.02.036

[101] Andreou I, Briasoulis A, Pappas C, et al. Ticagrelor versus Clopidogrel as part of dual or triple antithrombotic therapy: A systematic review and meta-analysis. Cardiovascular Drugs and Therapy. 2018;**32**:287-294. DOI: 10.1007/s10557-018-6795-9

[102] Kirolos I, Ifedili I, Maturana M, et al. Ticagrelor or prasugrel vs. clopidogrel in combination with anticoagulation for treatment of acute coronary syndrome in patients with atrial fibrillation. Annals of Translation Medicine. 2019;7:406. DOI: 10.21037/atm.2019.07.41

Chapter 4

Role of Medical Therapy in Chronic Mitral Regurgitation

Ruchika Meel

Abstract

Mitral regurgitation is one of the most commonly encountered valvular heart diseases in both the developing and the developed world. From various studies, it is known that chronic mitral regurgitation is associated with progressive left ventricular dysfunction, and eventually death if left untreated. This disease has a long silent period before symptoms manifest. During this latent period, left ventricular function progressively deteriorates and results in poor outcomes for patients even if surgery is performed. A few studies have evaluated the role of medical therapy in patients with chronic mitral regurgitation. This chapter will provide an overview of the use of medical therapy in chronic mitral regurgitation.

Keywords: chronic mitral regurgitation, medical therapy

1. Introduction

In heart failure (HF), irrespective of aetiology, there is activation of the sympathetic nervous system and the renin angiotensin system that initially serves as compensatory mechanism to maintain the falling cardiac output through retention of sodium and water, peripheral arterial vasoconstriction and increased cardiac contractility [1–3]. However, long term stimulation of these systems has a deleterious effect and results in cardiac remodelling and eventually irreversible HF in the absence of therapy [2, 4]. In HF due to chronic mitral regurgitation (MR) the aforementioned mechanisms are activated and over time result in apoptosis, necrosis and myocyte slippage and left ventricular (LV) remodelling and dilatation from loss of interstitial collagen [3]. There are a number of studies that have evaluated the effects of drugs in degenerative MR. Most of these involved beta blockers or vasodilators. The pathophysiologic basis for their use was to prevent the deleterious effect of sympathetic nervous system in MR, and medical therapy decreased afterload and LV wall stress, thus preventing deleterious remodelling [5].

In this review chapter a brief overview of aetiology and pathophysiology of MR will be provided, followed by the current perspective regarding the value of medical therapy in chronic MR will be discussed.

2. Definition and aetiology of mitral regurgitation

Chronic MR is a result of abnormality of the one or more of the components of the mitral valve apparatus [3, 6]. Mitral regurgitation can be a result of abnormality of mitral leaflet, chordae tendineae, papillary muscles and annulus. It can be

IntechOpen

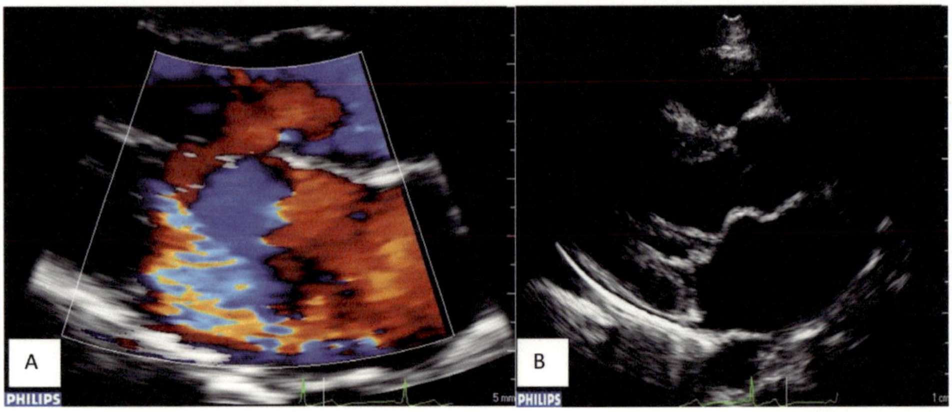

Figure 1.
(A) Parasternal long-axis view depicting an eccentric anteriorly directed mitral regurgitation jet secondary to restricted posterior mitral leaflet motion. (B) Parasternal long-axis view depicting a contemporary patient with established rheumatic heart disease: thickened shortened chordae, restricted posterior mitral leaflet [7].

primary or secondary. Primary MR is confined to de novo abnormality of the mitral leaflet itself, whereas secondary MR is as a result of another disease process usually involving the LV, which results in a regurgitant mitral valve. Mitral regurgitation results in volume overload of the LV and culminates in left ventricular failure if left untreated.

There are numerous aetiologies of mitral regurgitation [6]. The common cause of MR in the developed world is due to degenerative disease and in the developing world MR is due to rheumatic heart disease (**Figure 1**). Other causes of MR include: infective endocarditis, trauma, drugs, congenital heart disease and annular calcification. Secondary mitral regurgitation is due to coronary artery disease, cardiomyopathies (dilated, hypertrophic cardiomyopathy) and right ventricular pacing.

3. Pathophysiology of chronic mitral regurgitation

The amount of blood regurgitating into the left atrium depends on the size of the regurgitant orifice and the pressure gradient between the LV and the left atrium [3]. The regurgitant orifice and the gradient between the LV and the left atrium are not static. The pressure gradient between the two chambers is dependent on the peripheral vascular resistance. The mitral annulus is a dynamic structure and thus any change in the preload, afterload, and contractility alters the size of the annulus due to alteration the LV size. Therefore, when the afterload, preload and contractility decrease, the size of the mitral annulus decreases and so does the regurgitant orifice. Vasodilators, inotropes and diuretics tend to decrease the size of the LV, thus decreasing the mitral annulus size and the area of regurgitant orifice and hence the regurgitant volume. Conversely, any condition that increases the size of the LV increases the mitral annulus size and size of the regurgitant orifice. Further, in addition to magnitude of the pressure gradient difference the duration of the gradient has an effect on volume of regurgitation [8].

Thus, in summary the regurgitant volume can be estimated by the following formulae [9]:

Mitral Regurgitant Volume = Mitral Regurgitant Orifice Area × constant × Duration of pressure gradient × square root (LV Pressure – Left Atrial Pressure)

By altering the LV and left atrial pressure gradient and the orifice size various drugs can decrease or increase the mitral regurgitant volume.

Chronic MR is characterised by a compensated, transitional and decompensated stage [3, 10]. The compensated stage is characterised by LV remodelling. During this stage there is preserved ejection fraction as a result of eccentric ventricular hypertrophy accompanied by an elevated end diastolic volume. There is laying down of sarcomere in series and a shift in pressure-volume curve to the right with a larger volume for any given pressure. The transition phase is characterised by a decline in LV ejection fraction, the regurgitant volume and an increase in the afterload and there is a decrease in myocardial contractility. If untreated, the patient progresses into the decompensated state characterised by neurohormonal activation. There is increased LV stiffness with an increase in end-diastolic and end-systolic volume, preload and afterload with a decline in ejection fraction and stroke volume.

The compensated and the transition phase present opportunity for surgical intervention before the decompensated phase sets in and irreversible myocardial damages ensue. Current valvular heart disease guidelines recommend use of medical therapy for heart failure in patients with mitral regurgitation [11]. Medical therapy in the form of vasodilators and diuretics can be used in patients who are in decompensated phase and are at a high risk for surgery, and in the compensated phase where there is no indication for surgery. In the compensated phase the use of vasodilators aims to decrease the afterload, as it may help delay time to surgery [12].

4. Medical therapy in chronic mitral regurgitation

In chronic MR the persistent volume overload results in activation of compensatory mechanisms which include activation of sympathetic nervous system-renin angiotensin aldosterone system, the Frank-Starling mechanism and eccentric hypertrophy [3, 13]. Over the long-term, these compensatory mechanisms are deleterious and culminate in myocardial dysfunction and failure. These pathways have provided the rationale for benefit of medical therapy in MR. The following agents have been studied in chronic MR:

1. Vasodilators-angiotensin converting enzyme inhibitors (ACEI), angiotensin receptor blockers (ARB), hydralazine

2. Beta-blockers

3. Aldosterone receptor blockers

4. Combination anti-remodelling therapy

4.1 Vasodilators in chronic mitral regurgitation

Angiotensin converting enzyme inhibitors (ACEIs) and angiotensin receptor blockers (ARBs) reduce the severity of MR and hence HF symptoms by decreasing the afterload and potentially reversing the remodelling process. The decrease in predominantly peripheral vascular resistance results primarily in decrease in the size of the LV and thus size of the mitral annulus and that of the regurgitant orifice [14–16].

ACEIs have been used in the treatment of systolic HF with significant reductions in morbidity and mortality [17]. In the context of MR, benazepril was used in dogs with moderate to severe MR and showed improved survival [18]. Wisenbaugh et al. studied the effects of captopril in 32 patients with severe isolated MR over a 6-month period, and found no difference in LV diameters or ejection fraction when compared to placebo [19]. In a trial on humans assessing a combined population of patients with moderate to severe aortic regurgitation and MR, a significant reduction in regurgitant fraction, LV end-systolic and end diastolic volumes and LV mass, was noted when quinapril was used [20]. One study looked at the use of lisinopril in patients with chronic moderate MR with preserved LV ejection fraction and without symptoms. Twenty-three patients were randomised to receive lisinopril or placebo for a period of 12 months. A decrease in regurgitant fraction was noted in the group on lisinopril compared to the placebo arm without a change in left atrial or LV size [21].

In a paediatric case-control study of patients with moderate to severe MR the effect of ACEI on LV size and function was small after a follow-up period of 1 month to 1 year [22].

ARBs seem to produce a similar beneficial effect. In a, small study on the use of losartan for the treatment of MR, a modest but variable improvement in the severity of MR was noted. Specifically, the regurgitant volume and the effective regurgitant orifice decreased and the effect was durable for 1 month [15]. Another trial assessing moderate degenerative and rheumatic MR also found a beneficial effect with losartan over a 6-week period with regards to MR severity, LA size, and LV function [23].

Irbesartan was tested in an animal study. In this study irbesartan was administered to animals with new onset MR for a duration of 3 months. It reduced peripheral vascular resistance in the study group compared to group that received no therapy. However, no effect on LV dimensions was noted [24].

Hydralazine and lisinopril in combination with isosorbide dinitrate have been studied in patients with HF complicated by secondary MR [25, 26]. Hydralazine was tested in a small study of 15 patients with HF and MR, it should a variable response with half the patients showing no or minimal improvement over a follow-up period of 13 months. A second study looked at the benefit of lisinopril and isosorbide dinitrate in patients with HF and MR. This study showed an overall improvement in symptoms, hospitalisations due to HF and in peak oxygen consumption. In terms of reduction in MR severity and LV size, the response was variable.

It is important to note the aetiology of MR when using drugs that venodilate. Venodilators tend to worsen MR in patients with a fixed orifice such as rheumatic heart disease. In these patients venodilation results in a decrease in pulmonary venous pressure and hence a decrease in left atrial pressure, which results in tendency of the blood to follow the path of least resistance, that is, from LV into the left atrium. A reduction in just the systemic vascular resistance as in patients with rheumatic MR and co-morbidity of hypertension results in decrease in MR severity [26].

4.2 Beta blockers in chronic mitral regurgitation

The adrenergic system becomes activated at an early stage in patients with mitral regurgitation [27]. It acts as a support mechanism to maintain the contractility and cardiac output in MR. However, catecholamines are deleterious overlong term. Increased catecholamines induce myocyte apoptosis [28]. Hence, beta blockers are beneficial by preventing cardiac myocyte death due to excessive sympathetic activity.

Beta-blockade has demonstrated efficacy in reducing mortality in patients with cardiac failure due to non-valvular causes [17]. In canine models with chronic experimental MR chronic beta-blocker therapy improves LV function [13]. A pilot study involving patients with moderate to severe MR on beta-blocker therapy (metoprolol) was conducted over a 2-week period. Cardiac magnetic resonance imaging was used to follow-up this cohort. No reduction in regurgitant volume was demonstrated, however, LV work was reduced by beta-blocker therapy [29]. A larger study was therefore proposed to assess the effect of beta-blockers on LV function and symptoms due to MR. A subsequent trial was published, involving patients with moderate to severe, degenerative MR on beta-blocker therapy, (metoprolol) over a 2-year follow-up. LV function was assessed using cardiac magnetic resonance imaging. Improvements were found in LV ejection fraction and LV early diastolic filling rate. No change in LV end-diastolic volume or LV end-systolic volume was noted [30].

4.3 Aldosterone receptor antagonist in chronic mitral regurgitation

Aldosterone play an important role in HF progression [31]. In HF there is a decline in cardiac output which results in the activation of neurohormonal system and the renin angiotensin aldosterone pathway. The increased level of aldosterone stimulates inflammation and cardiac fibrosis. This results in pathologic cardiac remodelling.

Spironolactone has been evaluated in the context of systolic HF resulting in favourable LV remodelling and a decline in morbidity and mortality through aldosterone antagonism [17, 32]. The mortality reduction in HF was attributed to a decrease in sudden death and progression of HF. No human trials with spironolactone in MR have been noted in the literature. In dogs however, a study investigating spironolactone in moderate to severe MR resulted in a significant reduction (55%) in a composite end-point of cardiac-related death, euthanasia, or severe worsening of MR [33].

4.4 Combination anti-remodelling therapy in chronic mitral regurgitation

There is proven mortality and morbidity benefit of combination anti-remodelling therapy in systolic HF as a result of ischaemia and cardiomyopathies [17, 34, 35]. Guidelines on valvular heart disease recommend medical therapy for HF (EF < 50%) in chronic MR (class IIa, level of evidence B) [36]. However, there are no randomised controlled studies on effects of combination therapy in HF secondary to MR. Recently, in a small observational study Meel et al. showed that combination anti-remodelling therapy may be beneficial for HF secondary to chronic rheumatic MR with no HF related admissions or deaths, and no deterioration in echocardiographic parameters of ventricular size and function [37].

5. Conclusion

Most of above-mentioned trials were small studies involving vasodilators such as ACEIs and beta-blockers in degenerative MR and have been inconclusive. There is limited data pertaining to role of medical therapy in rheumatic MR. In general, LV dysfunction secondary to primary MR tends to respond poorly compared to LV dysfunction complicated by secondary MR. Currently there is no role of medical therapy in asymptomatic patients with chronic MR and preserved LV systolic function. Larger studies are needed to confirm benefit of medical therapy in chronic MR.

Conflicts of interest

The author has no conflicts of interest.

Funding

The author is the recipient of post-doctoral Carnegie Fellowship award.

Disclosures

Parts of this manuscript are a reproduction of author's own work on the subject of mitral regurgitation.

Author details

Ruchika Meel
Division of Cardiology, Department of Internal Medicine, University of the Witwatersrand, Johannesburg, Chris Hani Baragwanath Hospital, Johannesburg, South Africa

*Address all correspondence to: ruchikameel@gmail.com

References

[1] Hilfiker-Kleiner D, Landmesser U, Drexler H. Molecular mechanisms in heart failure focus on cardiac hypertrophy, inflammation, angiogenesis, and apoptosis. Journal of the American College of Cardiology. 2006;**48**:A56-A66

[2] Cohn J, Ferrari R, Sharpe N. Cardiac remodeling—Concepts and clinical implications: A consensus paper from an international forum on cardiac remodeling. Journal of the American College of Cardiology. 2000;**35**:569-582

[3] Bonow RO, Mann DL, Zipes DP, Libby P. Braunwald's Heart Disease. A Textbook of Cardiovascular Medicine. Vol. 9. Philadelphia: Elsevier Saunders; 2012

[4] Casaclang-Verzosa G, Gersh B, Tsang T. Structural and functional remodeling of the left atrium. Clinical and therapeutic implications for atrial fibrillation. Journal of the American College of Cardiology. 2008;**51**:1-11

[5] Carabello BA. The current therapy for mitral regurgitation. Journal of the American College of Cardiology. 2008;**52**:319-326

[6] Gaasch WH, Otto CM. Pathophysiology of Chronic Mitral Regurgitation. In: UpToDate, Post TW, editors. Waltham, MA: UpToDate; 2019

[7] Meel R et al. The changing spectrum of rheumatic mitral regurgitation in Soweto, South Africa. Cardiovascular Journal of Africa. 2017;**28**:215-220

[8] Topilsky Y, Michelena H, Bichara V, et al. Mitral valve prolapse with mid-late systolic mitral regurgitation: Pitfalls of evaluation and clinical outcome compared with holosystolic regurgitation. Circulation. 2012;**125**:1643

[9] Gaasch WH, Aurigemma GP. Inhibition of the renin-angiotensin system and the left ventricular adaptation to mitral regurgitation. Journal of the American College of Cardiology. 2002;**39**:1380

[10] Gaasch WH, Meyer TE. Left ventricular response to mitral regurgitation: Implications for management. Circulation. 2008;**118**:2298-2303

[11] Baumgartner H, Falk V, Bax JJ, De Bonis M, et al. ESC/EACTS guidelines for the management of valvular heart disease. European Heart Journal. 2017;**38**:2739-2791

[12] Gaasch WH, Otto CM. Vaosdilator Therapy in Chronic Mitral Regurgitation. In: UpToDate, Post TW, editors. Waltham, MA: UpToDate; 2018

[13] Tsutsui H, Spinale FG, Nagatsu M, et al. Effects of chronic beta-adrenergic blockade on the left ventricular and cardiocyte abnormalities of chronic canine mitral regurgitation. The Journal of Clinical Investigation. 1994;**93**:2639-2648

[14] Levine HJ, Gaasch WH. Vasoactive drugs in chronic regurgitant lesions of the mitral and aortic valves. Journal of the American College of Cardiology. 1996;**28**:1083

[15] Dujardin KS, Enriquez-Sarano M, Bailey KR, et al. Effect of losartan on degree of mitral regurgitation quantified by echocardiography. The American Journal of Cardiology. 2001;**87**:570

[16] Rosario LB, Stevenson LW, Solomon SD, et al. The mechanism of decrease in dynamic mitral regurgitation during heart failure treatment: Importance of reduction in the regurgitant orifice size. Journal of the American College of Cardiology. 1998;**32**:1819

[17] Yancy CW, Jessup M, Bozkurt B, et al. ACCF/AHA guideline for the management of heart failure: A report of the American College of Cardiology Foundation/American Heart Association task force on practice guidelines. Circulation. 2013;**128**:240-327

[18] Kittleson M, Rishniw M, Pion P, et al. Effect of benazepril on survival and cardiac events in dogs with asymptomatic mitral valve disease: A retrospective study of 141 cases. Journal of Veterinary Internal Medicine. 2009;**23**:953-954

[19] Wisenbaugh T, Sinovich V, Dullabh A, et al. Six month pilot study of captopril for mildly symptomatic, severe isolated mitral and isolated aortic regurgitation. The Journal of Heart Valve Disease. 1994;**3**:197-204

[20] Schön HR, Schröter G, Barthel P, et al. Quinapril therapy in patients with chronic mitral regurgitation. The Journal of Heart Valve Disease. 1994;**3**:303-312

[21] Marcotte F, Honos GN, Walling AD, et al. Effect of angiotensin-converting enzyme inhibitor therapy in mitral regurgitation with normal left ventricular function. The Canadian Journal of Cardiology. 1997;**13**:479

[22] Knirsch W, Tlach L, Stambach D, et al. Angiotensin-converting enzyme inhibitors in pediatric patients with mitral valve regurgitation—Case-control study and review of the literature. Congenital Heart Disease. 2010;**5**:278-284

[23] Sekuri C, Utuk O, Bayturan O, et al. Effect of losartan on exercise tolerance and echocardiographic parameters in patients with mitral regurgitation. Journal of the Renin-Angiotensin-Aldosterone System. 2008;**9**:107-111

[24] Perry GJ, Wei CC, Hankes GH, et al. Angiotensin II receptor blockade does not improve left ventricular function and remodeling in subacute mitral regurgitation in the dog. Journal of the American College of Cardiology. 2002;**39**:1374

[25] Greenberg BH, DeMots H, Murphy E, et al. Arterial dilators in mitral regurgitation: Effects on rest and exercise hemodynamics and long-term clinical follow-up. Circulation. 1982;**65**:181

[26] Levine AB, Muller C, Levine TB. Effects of high-dose lisinopril-isosorbide dinitrate on severe mitral regurgitation and heart failure remodeling. The American Journal of Cardiology. 1998;**82**:1299

[27] Carabello BA. Beta-blockade for mitral regurgitation. Could the management of valvular heart disease actually be moving into the 21st century? Journal of the American College of Cardiology. 2012;**60**:839-840

[28] Amin P, Singh M, Singh K. Adrenergic receptor-stimulated cardiac myocyte apoptosis: Role of 1 integrins. Journal of Signal Transduction. 2011:**2011**. Article ID: 179057

[29] Stewart S, Wilkinson W, Hansen C, et al. Predominance of heart failure in the heart of Soweto study cohort: Emerging challenges for Urban African communities. Circulation. 2008;**118**:2360-2367

[30] Ahmed M, Aban I, Lloyd S, et al. A randomized controlled phase IIb trial of beta 1-receptor blockade for chronic degenerative mitral regurgitation. Journal of the American College of Cardiology. 2012;**60**:833-838

[31] He BJ, Anderson ME. Aldosterone and cardiovascular disease: The heart of the matter. Trends in Endocrinology and Metabolism. 2013;**24**:21-30

[32] Soberman JE, Weber KT. Spironolactone in congestive heart

failure. Current Hypertension Reports. 2000;**2**:451-456

[33] Bernay F, Bland J, Häggström J, et al. Efficacy of spironolactone on survival in dogs with naturally occurring mitral regurgitation caused by myxomatous mitral valve disease. Journal of Veterinary Internal Medicine. 2010;**24**:331-341

[34] Merlo M, Pyxaras S, Pinamonti B, et al. Prevalence and prognostic significance of left ventricular reverse remodeling in dilated cardiomyopathy receiving tailored medical treatment. Journal of the American College of Cardiology. 2011;**57**:1468-1476

[35] Cicoira M, Zanolla L, Rossi A, et al. Long-term, dose-dependent effects of spironolactone on left ventricular function and exercise tolerance in patients with chronic heart failure. Journal of the American College of Cardiology. 2012;**40**:304-310

[36] Nishimura RA, Otto CM, Bonow RO, et al. AHA/ACC guideline for the management of patients with valvular heart disease: A report of the American College of Cardiology/ American Heart Association task force on practice guidelines. Journal of the American College of Cardiology. 2014;**63**:57-185

[37] Meel R, Peters F, Libhaber E, et al. Is there a role for combination anti-remodelling therapy for heart failure secondary to chronic rheumatic mitral regurgitation? Cardiovascular Journal of Africa. 2017;**28**:280

Section 2

Technical Aspect of Coronary Artery Bypass Grafting

Chapter 5

Coronary Artery Bypass Grafting: Surgical Anastomosis: Tips and Tricks

Mohd. Shahbaaz Khan

Abstract

The definite feature of coronary artery disease is the focal narrowing in the vascular endothelium, and this leads to the decrease in the flow of blood to the myocardium. Atherosclerotic plaque is the main lesion. These patients can present with chest pain (angina or myocardial infarction) and need further workup noninvasively and invasively for the management. The main reasons for myocardial revascularization can be: (1) relief from symptoms of myocardial ischemia; (2) reduce the risks of future mortality; (3) to treat or prevent morbidities such as myocardial infarction, arrhythmias, or heart failure. Coronary artery bypass grafting (CABG) is the surgical technique of cardiac revascularization. In 1910, Dr. Alexis Carrel described a series of canine experiments in which he devised means to treat CAD by creating a "complementary circulation" for the diseased native coronary arteries. No clinical translation occurred at the time, but he was awarded the Nobel Prize in Medicine. Experimental refinements of coronary arterial revascularization, including the use of internal thoracic artery (ITA) grafts, were later reported by Murray and colleagues, Demikhov, and Goetz and colleagues in the 1950s and early 1960s. Dr. Rene Favaloro performed his first coronary bypass operation in May 1967 with an interposed saphenous vein graft (SVG) and shortly thereafter used aortocoronary bypasses sutured proximally to the ascending aorta. The stenosed segment is bypassed using an arterial or venous graft. Left internal thoracic artery is the most commonly used artery, and long saphenous vein is the most commonly used vein for the coronary artery grafting to reestablish the blood flow to the compromised myocardium. This can be performed with or without the help of cardiopulmonary bypass machine and also with or without arresting the heart. These techniques are called as on-pump beating or on-pump arrested and off-pump beating coronary artery bypass grafting surgery. Distal and proximal anastomoses are usually performed in an end-to-side manner, but in the case of doing sequential grafting, side-to-side anastomosis is also performed proximal to the end-to-side anastomosis. In this chapter we are going to discuss the coronary artery bypass grafting tips and tricks in details.

Keywords: coronary artery bypass grafting, off-pump CABG, on-pump CABG, LIMA, RIMA, radial, RSVG, sequential grafting

1. Introduction

Coronary artery disease is a major cause of mortality and morbidity not only in the developed countries but also in developing countries. Over the last decade,

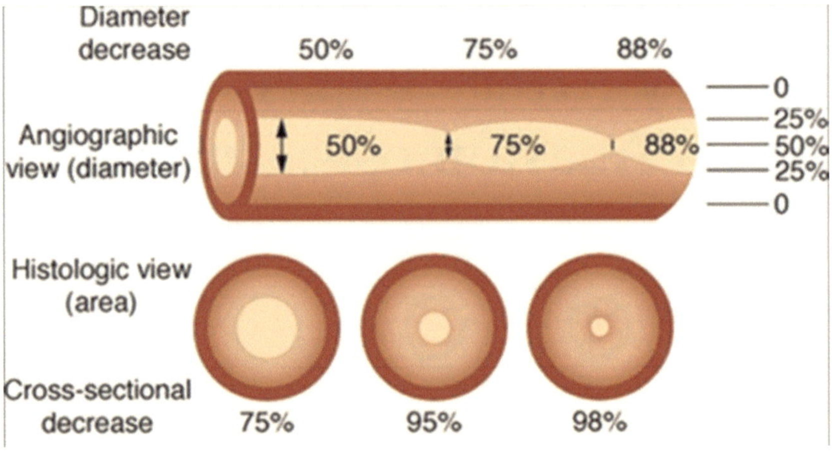

Figure 1.
Relationship between loss of cross-sectional area and diameter of the vessel.

mortality with this disease has decreased, but still it accounts for approximately one-third of all the deaths in people over the age of 35 years. The American Heart Association reported that nearly 16.5 million people (20 years or more age) had coronary artery disease in 2017, with male predominance of 55% [1].

Coronary artery disease is the narrowing or occlusion of the vessel lumen due to arterial wall thickening caused by subintimal deposition of atheroma and loss of elasticity of the arterial wall. Atherosclerosis involves the proximal portions of the coronary arteries, specifically at the branching sites. In the beginning it only affects the flow reserve of the coronary artery, but as it advances, it affects the blood flow even at rest and leads to myocardial ischemia or infarction depending on the severity of the disease. This can be divided as supply ischemia (myocardial infarction and unstable angina) and demand ischemia (stable angina as during exercise, fever, emotional stress, etc.) [2]. The subendocardium is most vulnerable to myocardial ischemia due to the limited collateral blood flow. Therefore myocardial necrosis progresses from the subendocardium to the epicardium with continuing ischemia.

A 75% cross-sectional area loss (50% diameter) is considered an important but moderate stenosis, while a 90% cross-sectional area loss (67% diameter) is considered severe stenosis (**Figure 1**) [3].

There are three methods of treating coronary artery disease—medical management, percutaneous intervention, and coronary artery bypass graft surgery [4, 5].

2. Medical management of coronary artery disease

1. Aspirin—it should be used daily in the case of stable angina. Daily use of aspirin in stable angina decreases myocardial infarction and sudden death. Its role is very important in unstable angina and myocardial infarction. Aspirin should also be continued after PCI or CABG.

2. Platelet inhibitors—it inhibits the binding of the ADP to platelet P2Y12 receptors and consequently inhibits activation of GPIIb/IIIa complex. Therefore it inhibits platelet aggregation. Clopidogrel is recommended if patient is intolerable to aspirin or there are adverse or side effects of aspirin such as GI bleeding or allergic reaction [6]. Both aspirin and clopidogrel are

recommended for at least 1 year after PCI and CABG. Aspirin and clopidogrel combination is not recommended for stable angina as it is not superior to aspirin alone and increases the risk of bleeding [7].

3. Beta blockers—these medicines decrease the myocardial oxygen demand and improve exercise capacity. These are effective for stable angina, and dose should be adjusted to keep heart rate about 60/min at rest and less than 100/min with exercise.

4. Calcium channel blocker—as beta blockers, these agents are also effective to treat stable angina. They act mainly by causing vasodilatation and reducing peripheral vascular resistance. The dihydropyridines (nifedipine, amlodipine, etc.) do not affect the SA or AV node conduction. Their mechanism of action is by dilating the coronary arteries and reducing the peripheral residence, thereby leading to the decrease in myocardial oxygen demand. On the other hand, non-dihydropyridines (verapamil, diltiazem, etc.) also affect the SA and AV nodes and decrease the oxygen demand.

5. Nitrates—these are the coronary vasodilator agents. In the lower doses, they are venodilator and reduce the preload, while in higher doses they are also arterial dilators and thereby decrease the afterload too.

6. Ranolazine—this is the selective inhibitor of the late influx of sodium, thus decreasing the myocardial contractility. It is usually used in combination with beta blockers to treat angina.

7. Statins—these are hypolipidemic drugs that inhibit the HMG-CoA reductase enzyme and decrease atherosclerotic effect.

8. ACE inhibitors—they inhibit the angiotensin-converting enzyme. These are the class I recommendation for patients with chronic coronary artery disease with low LVEF (<40%) or diabetic and a class II recommendation for patients without these mentioned features [8].

3. Percutaneous coronary intervention (PCI)

Although the term percutaneous coronary intervention refers to any therapeutic coronary artery intervention, it has become synonymous with the percutaneous coronary stent implantation. In the earlier days, bare metal stents were used, but over the last decades, drug-eluting stents are the most commonly used stents for PCI. PCI is performed in patients with stable coronary artery disease and also in settings of acute coronary syndrome.

3.1 Indications for PCI

1. Moderate to severe stable angina with evidence of reversible ischemia.

2. High-risk unstable angina or ST elevation myocardial infarction (STEMI).

3. Acute STEMI.

4. Rescue PCI after failed thrombolysis.

5. Cardiogenic shock after myocardial infarction (MI).

6. Revascularization after successful resuscitation.

3.2 Absolute contraindication

1. Lack of vascular access.

2. Active untreatable severe bleeding.

3.3 Relative contraindications

1. Bleeding disorder.

2. Severe renal insufficiency unless patient is on hemodialysis or has severe electrolyte abnormality.

3. Sepsis.

4. Poor compliance with medicines.

5. Terminal illness (advanced or metastatic malignancy).

6. Short life expectancy.

7. Difficult coronary anatomy.

8. Failed previous PCI or not amenable to PCI.

9. Severe cognitive dysfunction or advanced physical limitation.

10. Other indication for open heart surgery.

3.4 In view of the following conditions, patients should not go for PCI

1. Small area of myocardium is at risk.

2. No objective evidence of ischemia with either noninvasive or invasive testing (e.g., fractional flow reserve).

3. Less likelihood of technical success.

4. Left main coronary artery (LM) or multivessel coronary artery disease with a high SYNTAX score (better for CABG).

5. Insignificant stenosis ($<$50% stenosis).

6. End-stage cirrhosis with portal hypertension resulting in encephalopathy or visceral bleeding.

4. Coronary artery bypass grafting (CABG)

Coronary artery bypass grafting is a coronary revascularization by surgery. Dr Rene Favaloro performed his first coronary bypass operation in May 1967 with an interposed saphenous vein graft (SVG) and shortly thereafter used aortocoronary bypasses sutured proximally to the ascending aorta. In the words of Dr Denton Cooley, "Although he [Favaloro] was always hesitant to carry the moniker of 'father' of coronary artery bypass surgery, he is the surgeon we should credit with introducing coronary bypass surgery into the clinical arena" [9]. It has been shown to be highly effective in the relief of severe angina and under some circumstances has the capability for considerably prolonging useful life. The stenosed segment of the coronary artery is bypassed using an arterial or venous conduit, and by this it reestablishes the blood flow to the distal ischemic myocardial area. Many studies have shown that surgical revascularization is superior to medical and percutaneous interventional management for multivessel CAD. Full workup should be done before taking patient for surgery.

4.1 The anatomical factors which favor the CABG are as follows

1. Significant LM disease.

2. Significant proximal left anterior descending (LAD) disease.

3. Lesions not amenable to PCI.

4. Diabetes mellitus.

5. Depressed left ventricular (LV) ejection fraction.

Indications for CABG can be classified as per **Table 1**.

4.2 Indications for CABG

1. High-grade LM stenosis.

2. Significant stenosis (>75%) of proximal LAD with double- or triple-vessel disease.

Treatment Class	Description
I	Conditions for which the operation is indicated on the basis of a demonstrated advantage over medical treatment in terms of longevity or relief of symptoms or both
II	Conditions for which the operation is acceptable treatment but for which its advantages over medical treatment have not yet been fully defined
III	Conditions for which the operation is not generally considered to be indicated, because of lack of demonstrated advantage over medical treatment.

Table 1.
Classification of indications for CABG surgery.

3. Symptomatic double- or triple-vessel disease.
4. Disabling angina despite maximal medical therapy.
5. Poor LV functions.
6. Post MI angina.
7. Post NSTEMI with ongoing ischemia that is unresponsive to medical therapy or PCI.
8. STEMI with inadequate response to all nonsurgical management.
9. Emergency CABG.
10. Failed PCI.

4.3 Contraindications

4.3.1 Absolute contraindication

There is no absolute contraindication.

4.3.2 Relative contraindications

1. Asymptomatic patient with low risk of MI or death.
2. Advanced age.
3. Co-morbidities (COPD, pulmonary hypertension, etc.)

4.4 Factors increasing mortality after CABG

1. Preoperative renal insufficiency.
2. Peripheral vascular disease.
3. Recent MI.
4. Recent brain stroke.
5. Emergency surgery.
6. Cardiogenic shock.

5. Types of grafts

5.1 Arterial grafts

- Internal thoracic artery (internal mammary artery)
- Radial artery

- Right gastroepiploic artery
- Inferior epigastric artery
- Ulnar artery
- Splenic artery

5.2 Venous grafts

- Greater saphenous vein
- Short saphenous vein
- Cephalic vein

5.3 Arterial grafts

5.3.1 Left internal mammary artery (LIMA)/left internal thoracic artery (LITA)

Drs. Vineberg and Miller were the first to recognize the properties of internal mammary artery (IMA) and used it for myocardial revascularization in 1945 [10]. They found that it is usually spared from atherosclerosis and reasoned that its branches could form collaterals with myocardial arterioles. They injected contrast medium in postmortem specimens demonstrating connections between the implant and the coronary arteries, but few surgeons took their work seriously [11].

LIMA originates from subclavian artery just above and behind the sternal end of the clavicle (**Figure 2**). The artery descends vertically 1 cm lateral to the sternal border, behind the first six costal cartilages. **Figure 3** shows the LIMA position regarding pectoralis muscle, sternum, and pleura with endothoracic fascia. LIMA is widely used these days, especially for the anastomosis with LAD. After dividing the sternum, retractor is placed to lift the left sterna edge. The operating table can be elevated and rotated to expose LIMA properly and harvest it. LIMA can be harvested as pedicle graft (along with internal thoracic veins, fat, muscles, and pleura) or skeletonized vessel. Skeletonized LIMA is supposed to preserve the venous drainage of the sternum, and it is often preferred when there is suspicion of sternal healing and wound infection. All small branches of LIMA are clipped. The proximal end of the LIMA kept attached to the subclavian artery, and then after giving heparin, the distal end is ligated and divided. In the same way as LIMA is harvested, RIMA can also be harvested if it is needed for grafting.

5.3.2 Radial artery

The second most commonly used artery is the radial artery (RA). It is usually harvested from nondominant hand (**Figure 4**). The RA arises from the bifurcation of the brachial artery in the cubital fossa and terminates by forming the deep palmar arch in the hand. The main concern using RA is blood supply to the wrist and hand. Before using the radial artery, we should assess the patency and collateral blood circulation from the ulnar artery. It can be assessed clinically by Allen's and modified Allen's tests. This can also be assessed by preoperative arterial ultrasound.

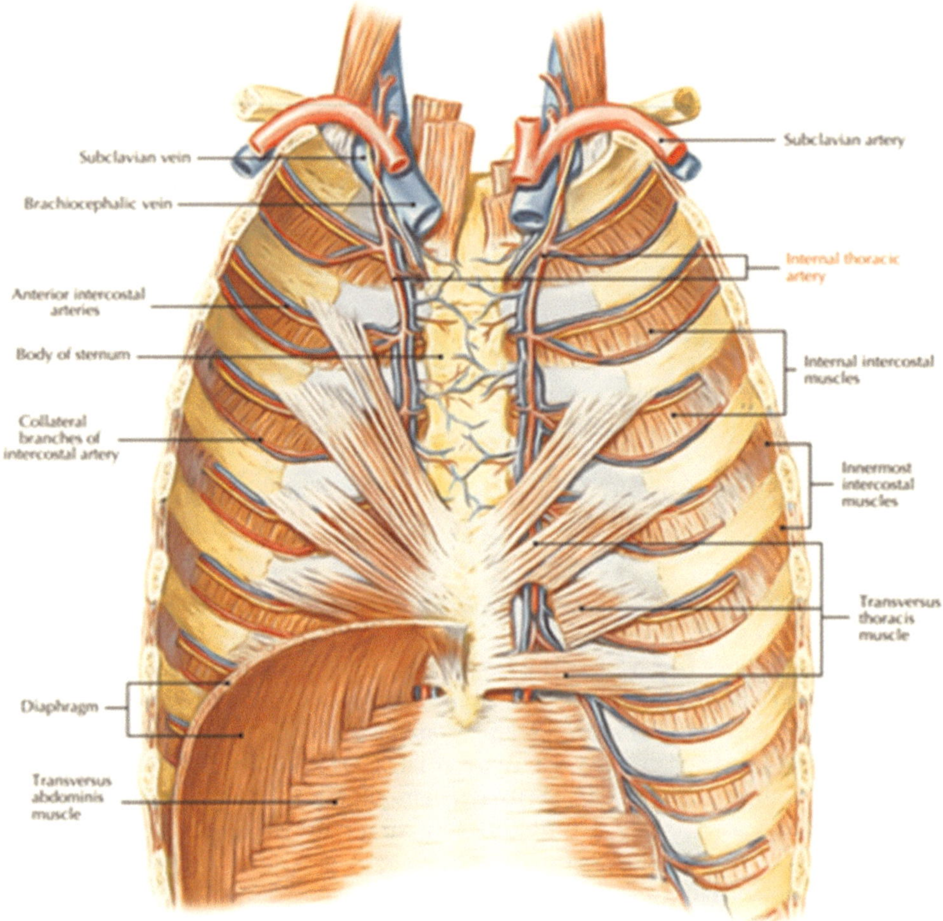

Figure 2.
Internal mammary artery course.

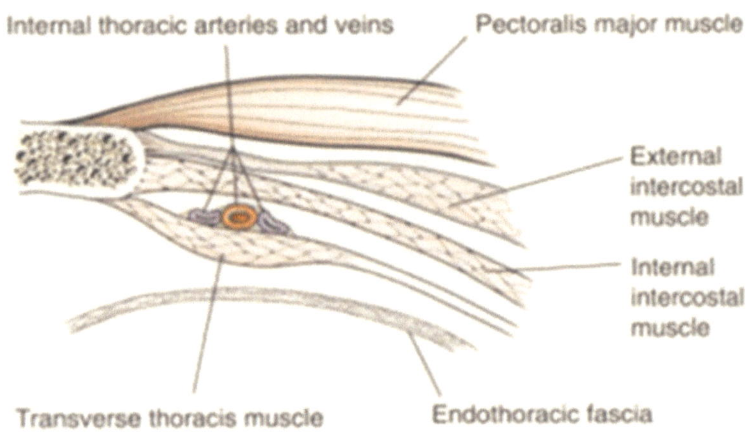

Figure 3.
Relationship of LIMA with sternum, thoracic muscles, pleura, and endothoracic fascia.

The radial artery can be harvested by open conventional method or endoscopically. The radial artery should be flushed and kept in a solution prepared with Ringer lactate (500 ml), sodium nitroprusside (50 mg), and heparinized blood (30 ml).

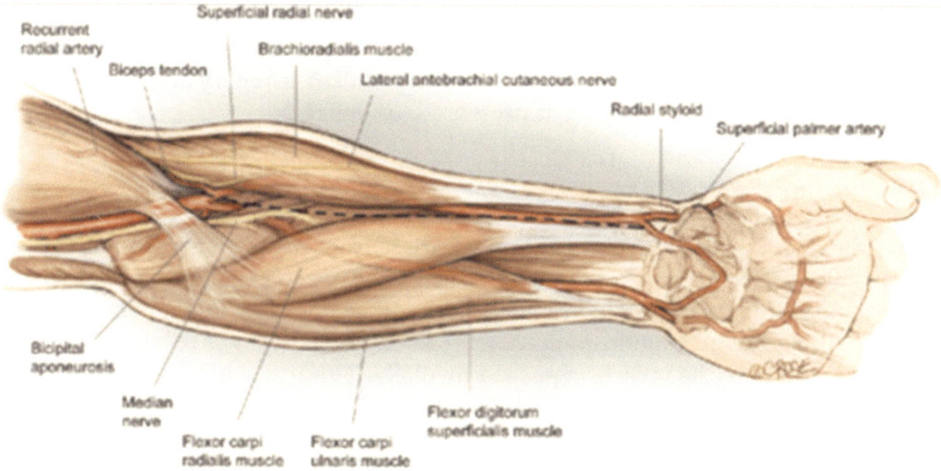

Figure 4.
Radial artery and palmer arch.

5.3.3 Right gastroepiploic artery

It is very rarely used as an arterial graft when other conduits are not available. To harvest this artery, the midline incision over the sternum is extended to the upper abdomen, and the abdominal cavity is opened. There are two gastroepiploic arteries (**Figure 5**): left and right. Both arteries participate in the stomach vascularization and are collateral blood circulation with other blood vessels of the stomach. Harvesting right gastroepiploic artery as conduit does not compromise stomach blood supply. Branches of this artery to the stomach and omentum are ligated and divided. This artery is positioned either anteriorly or posteriorly to the duodenum

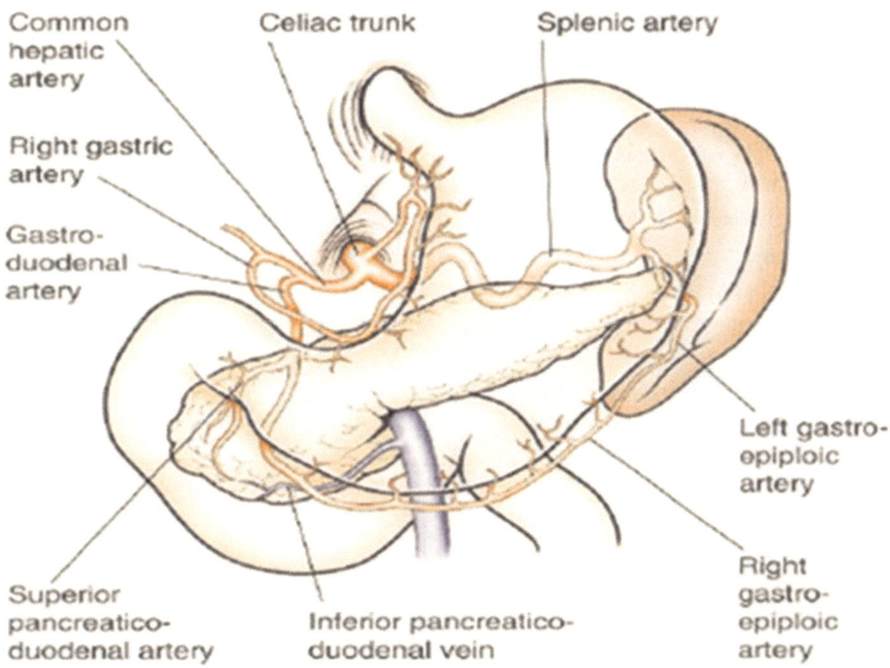

Figure 5.
Gastroepiploic artery.

and stomach, depending on the tension on graft. A circular opening is made in the diaphragm, medial to the inferior vena cava, and the gastroepiploic artery is passed through this opening to anastomose it with RCA or PDA coronary arteries. The anatomy of gastroepiploic arteries is presented in **Figure 6**.

5.3.4 Inferior epigastric artery

The inferior epigastric artery (**Figure 6**) arises from the medial aspect of the external iliac artery and gives branches to the spermatic cord, pubis, abdominal muscles, and skin. Its harvesting requires additional either low midline, or paramedian, or oblique inguinal approach. The anterior sheath of the rectus muscle is divided, and then the muscle is pushed medially. The artery is harvested along with the accompanying veins as a pedicle graft and kept in the solution as mentioned for radial artery preservation.

When the length of this artery is not sufficient for an independent graft, it is used as a composite graft with the LIMA as extension graft.

5.3.5 Ulnar artery

Occasionally, when surgeons do not have other choice, they use the ulnar artery as arterial conduit.

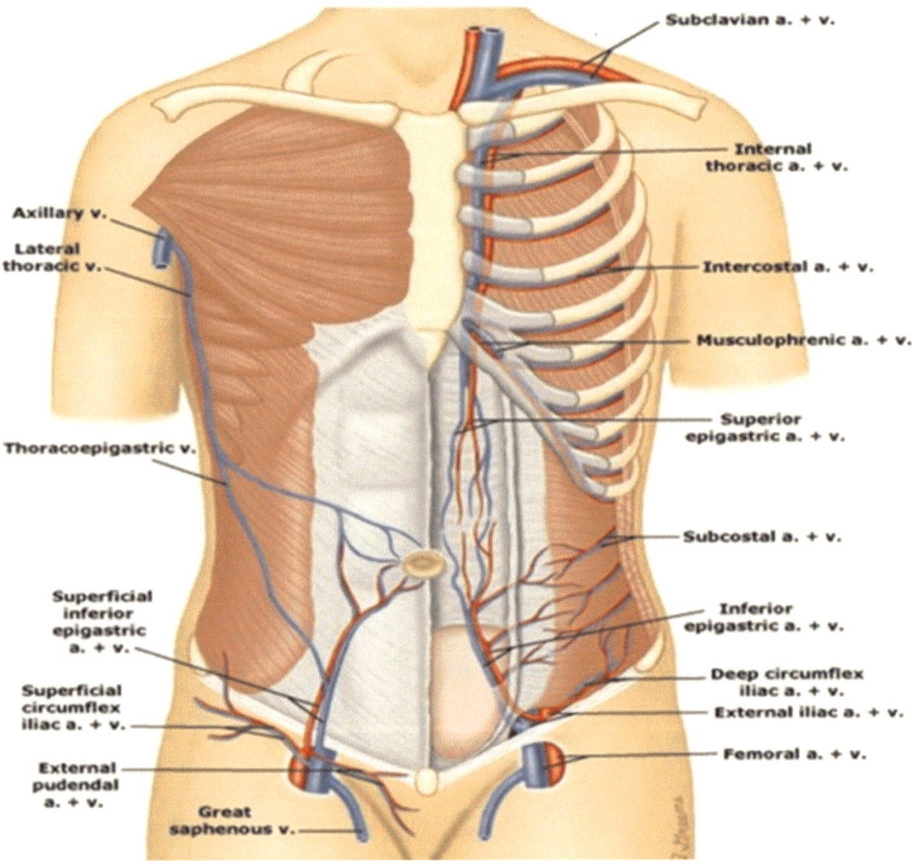

Figure 6.
Inferior epigastric artery.

5.3.6 Splenic artery

When there is lack of other conduit, the splenic artery can be used for grafting. The same as harvesting gastroepiploic artery, midline sternal incision can be extended over the abdomen, and the abdomen is opened. Then lesser peritoneal sac is opened. The splenic artery (**Figure 7**) runs along the superior margin of the pancreas. Branches to the pancreas are ligated and divided. Then the splenic artery is ligated and divided at the splenic hilum and passed through an opening made in the diaphragm medial to the inferior vena cava.

5.4 Venous grafts

5.4.1 Greater saphenous vein

The greater saphenous vein (**Figure 8**) is the most commonly used conduit for CABG. The greater saphenous vein (GSV) of the lower extremity is the best choice of this type of graft based on:

- There are two independent types of low extremity vein system, and removal of superficial one (GSV) does not jeopardize the venous flow from the leg.

- Position, diameter, and length of the GSV are in constant pattern which simplifies its harvest.

Usually a single long segment is harvested. About 12–15 cm segment may be needed for diagonal branch, about 20–24 cm length for OM branches, and 18–22 cm

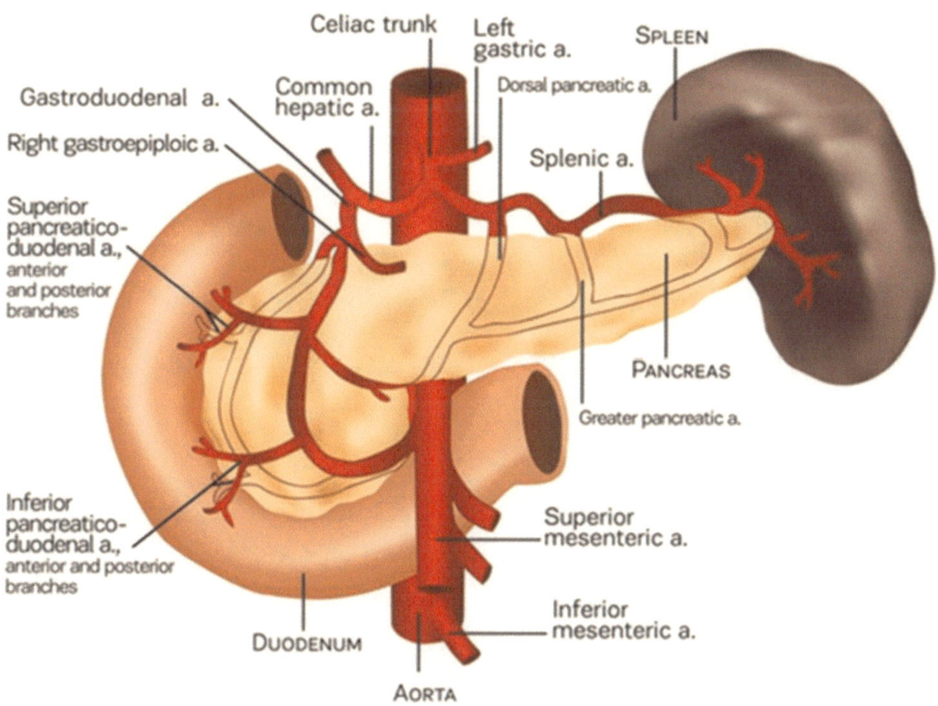

Figure 7.
Splenic artery.

length for RCA and PDA coronary arteries. Poor quality and veins with varicosities should be avoided. Branches can either be ligated or clipped. These should be ligated or clipped; just flush with GSV to avoid the narrowing or diverticulum. Creation of skin flaps should also be avoided.

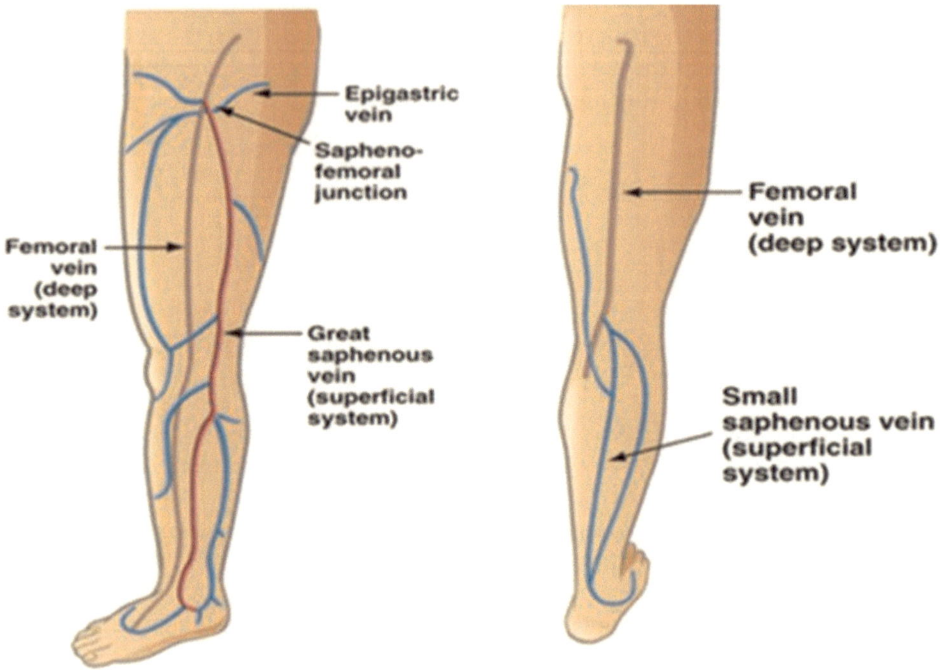

Figure 8.
Greater and short saphenous veins.

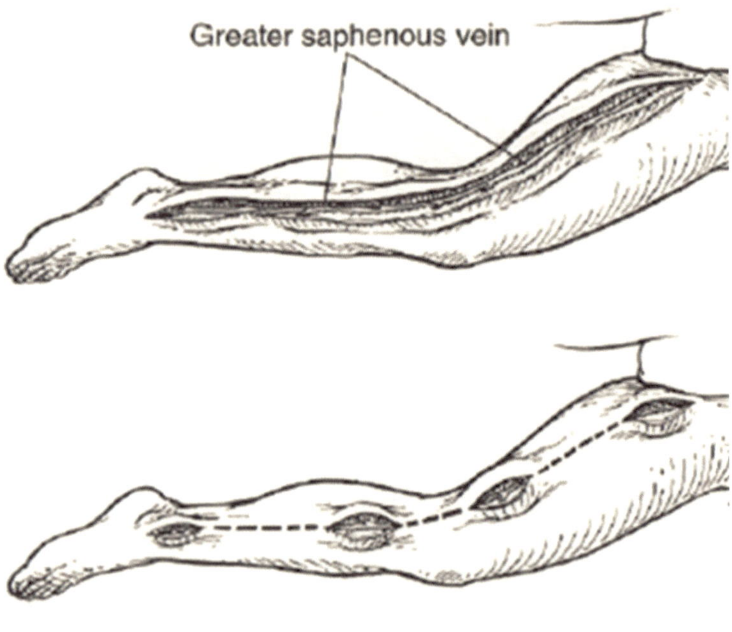

Figure 9.
Direct continuous and interrupted harvesting method of SVG.

GSV is harvested in two different ways:

- Directly by single full incision or through multiple incisions (**Figure 9**)
- Endoscopic vein harvest

5.4.2 Short saphenous vein

In rare cases when not enough conduits are available, some surgeons have to use short saphenous vein (**Figure 8**). It can be harvested by positioning the patient in prone or supine position.

5.4.3 Cephalic vein

Even though we have not used the vein as alternative graft, this can be used in the case other grafts need it. The cephalic vein can be harvested from the wrist up to the shoulder. The walls of the vein are thinner than the saphenous veins, and long-term patency is also lesser than saphenous veins [12].

6. Types of CABG

1. Traditional on-pump CABG.
2. Off-pump CABG.
3. Minimally invasive direct.
4. Totally endoscopic CABG.

6.1 On-pump CABG technique

- A median sternotomy is done (**Figure 10**).
- The same time arterial or venous conduit is harvested.
- LIMA is harvested.
- Full-dose heparin is given.
- LIMA is divided distally and a bulldog clamp is placed on the artery.
- Distal segment of LIMA on the chest wall is ligated or clipped.
- The pericardium is opened and pericardial stay sutures placed.
- Purse string sutures are placed on the ascending aorta and right atrial appendage for cannulation.
- A purse string suture is placed on the ascending aorta for cardioplegia cannulation.
- Aortic and right atrial cannulae are inserted.

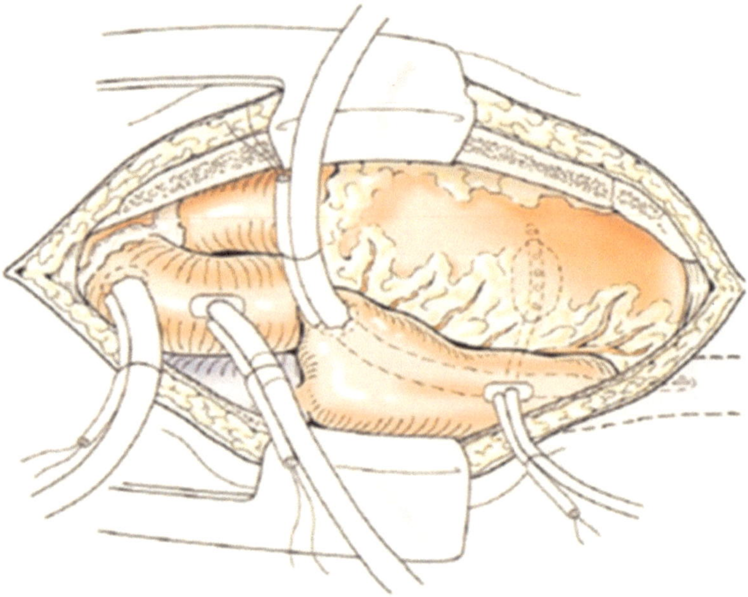

Figure 10.
Cannulation for on-pump CABG.

- Epiaortic ultrasound can be used to find the site devoid of calcification or atherosclerotic plaques, for cannulation [13].

- Aorta is cross clamped and antegrade cardioplegia given.

- Cold saline or ice slush can be used for topical cooling.

- The heart is retracted out of the pericardial cavity, toward the head of the patient.

- Usually first distal graft is done to RCA or PDA (**Figure 11**).

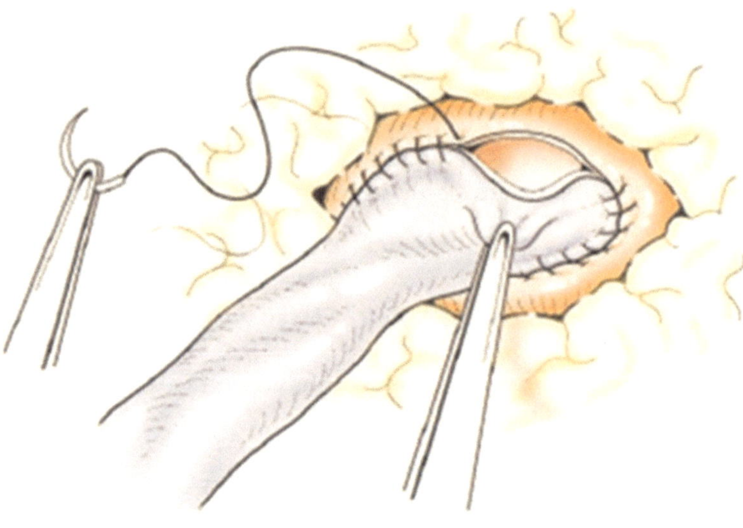

Figure 11.
SVG-coronary artery anastomosis.

- Graft is distended with blood cardioplegic solution, graft lie is checked, and appropriate length is divided.
- The heart is then retracted to the right and then OM is selected for grafting.
- Distal anastomosis is done to selected OM vessel.
- Graft is distended with solution and appropriate length divided.
- The same technique is used for diagonal anastomosis.
- Then focus is changed to LIMA-LAD anastomosis.
- LIMA is cut to appropriate length.
- LIMA-LAD anastomosis is created with Polypropylene 7-0 or 8-0 sutures (**Figure 12**).
- Rewarming is started while doing anastomosis.
- A pericardial window is made to pass LIMA without tension.
- Phrenic nerve should not be injured.
- Aortic cross clamp is removed.
- Partially occluding clamp is applied on the ascending aorta (**Figure 13**).
- Two to three openings are made in the aorta using aortic punch.
- Proximal anastomosis is done between the aorta and grafts with Prolene 6-0 sutures.
- Partially occluding clamp is removed.
- De-airing of the grafts is done.

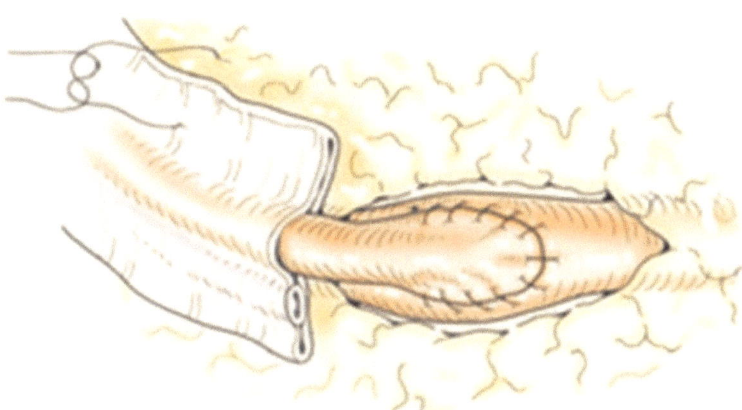

Figure 12.
LIMA-LAD anastomosis.

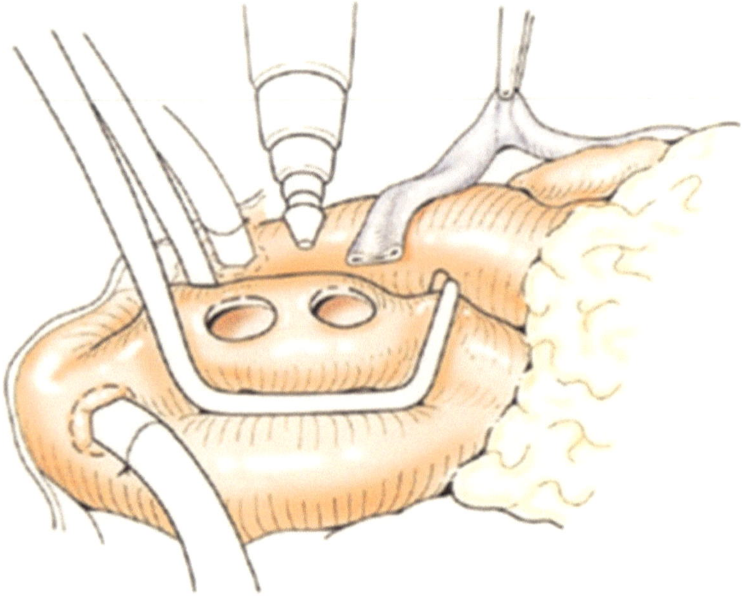

Figure 13.
Side-biting clamp on the ascending aorta for proximal anastomosis.

- Proximal anastomosis can also be done on the arrested heart with single aortic cross clamp [14],
- If the heart is in sinus rhythm, then start weaning off CPB.
- Graft flow could be checked with flow meter device.
- Protamine is given to reverse the effect of heparin.
- Decannulation is done and bleeding secured.
- Temporary pacing wire is placed on RV.
- One mediastinal and one left pleural drains are inserted.
- Sternum is closed with wires.
- The skin and subcutaneous tissue are closed in layers with vicryl sutures.

6.2 Off-pump CABG (OPCABG) technique

6.2.1 Patient selection

6.2.1.1 Beginner beating heart surgeon

They should avoid patients with unfavorable characteristics:

- Cardiomegaly-making exposure of lateral and inferior walls difficult
- Small (<1.5 mm diameter), intramyocardial, and diffusely diseased vessels

- Hemodynamically unstable patients
- Critical left main disease
- Recent acute MI
- LV EF <35%

6.2.1.2 Experienced beating heart surgeons

Majority of the cases can be performed without complication after getting a good experience in off-pump CABG, but it is better to avoid if multiple unfavorable factors are present in the same patient (cardiomegaly with EF <25% and small vessels).

OPCAB is particularly beneficial for:

- High-risk patients
- Left ventricle dysfunction
- High calcific load
- Age older than 75 years
- Diabetes mellitus
- Renal failure
- Left main stem disease
- Reoperations
- Chronic pulmonary disease
- An overall EuroSCORE >5 [15, 16]

6.3 Contraindications

6.3.1 Absolute contraindications

- Preoperative hemodynamic instability
- Deep myocardial LAD
- Moderate to severe mitral regurgitation

6.3.2 Relative contraindications

- Pulmonary hypertension
- Diffuse coronary artery disease
- Dense myocardial adhesions during reoperative surgery

- Enlarged ascending aorta
- LM disease with a non-reconstructable RCA system

6.4 Operative steps

- Preserve normothermia by keeping the operating room warm.
- CPB machine and perfusionist should be available in OR.
- No need to prime the CPB machine.
- Off-pump setup (octopus, starfish, CO_2 blower, intracoronary shunts) should also be available (**Figure 14**).
- Maintaining the systolic BP is important during positioning of the heart for grafting.
- Inotropic supports and IV fluid is usually required.
- Midline sternotomy.
- LIMA and other conduits are harvested.
- Heparin is given (1–1.5 mg/Kg) to keep ACT of about 300 s.
- ACT should be checked every 20 min and added as required.
- Coronary arteries should be grafted in the order of increasing cardiac displacement (anterior wall vessels, then inferior wall, and finally lateral wall vessels).

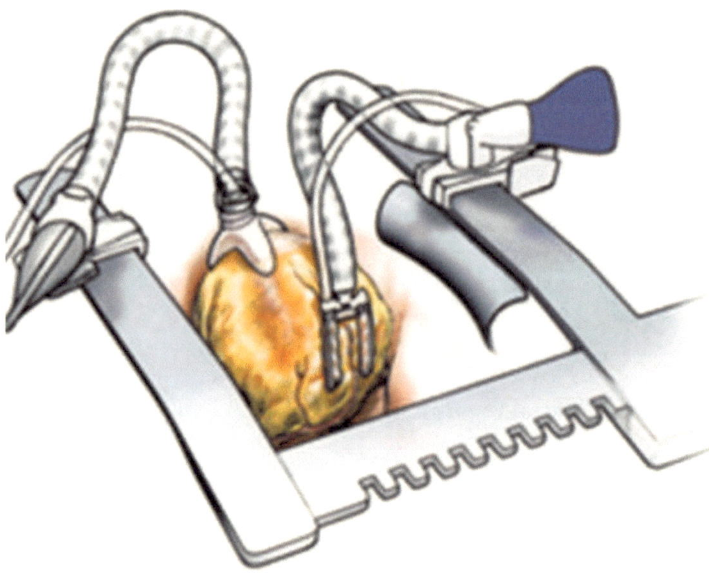

Figure 14.
OPCABG setup: octopus and starfish.

DOI: http://dx.doi.org/10.5772/intechopen.88932

- Most of the surgeons usually do distal anastomoses first, but proximal anastomoses can be done before distal anastomoses.

- Performing proximal aortic anastomoses last allows precise estimation of graft length, whereas performing them first allows immediate myocardial reperfusion once each distal anastomosis is completed.

- Positioning the heart is very important and needs mechanical stabilizers as octopus and starfish.

- **Anterior wall vessel anastomosis**—anterior wall vessels (LAD, diagonal, ramus) need to be brought near midline for better visualization and anastomosis. Deep pericardial retraction sutures of silk, vicryl, or ethibond (1-0) should be taken fast near the left superior pulmonary vein in order to prevent hemodynamic instability.

- **Inferior wall vessel anastomosis**—for distal right coronary artery and posterior descending artery, the table is in steep Trendelenburg position. Manipulation of the deep pericardial retraction sutures is done to better expose the grafting vessel. For grafting the right coronary artery, the table is made flat, and retraction sutures are relaxed with the heart failing to the left side. Maneuvering the heart for RCA and PDA grafting can cause bradycardia and hypotension, so anesthetists should be more vigilant and need to give fluid and inotropes to keep hemodynamic stability during grafting.

- **Lateral wall vessel anastomosis**—for obtuse marginals, posterolateral branches of the right coronary artery, the OR table is placed in steep Trendelenburg position, raised and rotated toward the right [17]. This will allow gravity to displace the heart to the right and apex anteriorly. The right pleura is opened, and the right pericardial incision is extended toward the inferior vena cava, so that the heart can be displaced toward the right side without hemodynamic compromise. Some extra deep pericardial retraction sutures may need to be taken between the inferior vena cava and pulmonary vein. The first suture is anchored just above the left superior pulmonary vein, the second below the left inferior pulmonary vein, the third one called "the intermediate" is located between the inferior pulmonary vein and the inferior vena cava, and the fourth one close to the inferior vena cava. These stitches are quite comparable to the "Lima Stitches" introduced in North America in 1997 by Tom Salerno [18].

- Do not compromise the exposure, and if it is not possible, then convert to conventional on-pump CABG.

- A silastic tape or vascular sling is passed around the selected coronary artery proximal to the site chosen for anastomosis.

- Intracoronary shunts are inserted in coronary arteriotomy.

- A CO2 blower is used to disperse the blood to create the anastomosis.

- Blower is used selectively when needed and at a rate not >5 L/min to prevent endothelial damage.

- A temporary pacing wire can be placed for anastomosis to RCA to combat the bradycardia.
- Anastomosis is performed in a routine manner with Polypropylene 7-0 or 8-0 sutures for LIMA grafting or venous grafting.
- The intima of both the graft and the recipient vessels must be visualized each time the needle is placed through the anastomosis.
- Bilateral IMA grafting (typically to the left heart) has been shown to improve survival and intervention-free survival and should be performed whenever contraindications do not exist.
- After completion of anastomoses, heparin could be reversed with protamine.
- Protamine is given (0.75–1.0 mg/kg) to incompletely reverse the heparin, leaving each patient with an ACT less than 150 s at the conclusion of the case.
- The avoidance of CPB should not come at the price of any compromise in anastomotic precision.

6.5 Hemodynamic instability and conversion to cardiopulmonary bypass

In some of the situations, CABG should be performed on CPB. These are as follows:

a. Ischemic arrhythmias unresponsive to heparin and antiarrhythmic medications.

b. Cardiogenic shock due to acute infarction or severe global ischemia.

c. Physical conditions that limit rightward displacement of the heart (deep pectus excavatum, previous left pneumonectomy)

Although avoidance of CPB is generally a worthwhile goal, it does not supersede the goals of hemodynamic stability and complete, precise revascularization.

6.6 Causes of hemodynamic instability

- Imperfect technique in cardiac displacement (compressing the right atrium or right ventricle or kinking of the right ventricular outflow tract during rightward displacement of the heart).
- Application of compression with the coronary stabilizer—achieve and maintain tissue capture with a minimum of downward pressure on the heart. This will optimize both coronary stabilization and hemodynamic stability.
- Less commonly, regional myocardial ischemia is a cause of hemodynamic instability.

The risk of myocardial ischemia during off-pump CABG can be reduced by keeping the following points in consideration:

- The most stenotic vessel is always revascularized first because this vessel is normally well collateralized.
- The proximal anastomosis of the graft is performed just after the distal anastomosis of the same graft is completed before proceeding to the next distal anastomosis.
- Intracoronary shunts are used to prevent ischemia.
- The ascending aorta is side clamp only once during the procedure to minimize the aortic trauma.
- The systemic pressure is always reduced around 90–100 mmHg before and during the entire side clamping of the ascending aorta.
- The anterior and the inferior territories are always grafted before the posterior territory.

6.7 Sequential bypass grafting

The sequential bypass graft is an effective multiple-bypass technique when graft availability is limited [19] and has been reported to allow improved rates of patency in bypass procedures on narrow coronary arteries [20, 21]. Compared with regular end-to-side anastomosis, however, side-to-side anastomosis is a relatively complex procedure.

Methods of side-to-side anastomosis include the following:

1. A diamond configuration, in which the graft axis lies perpendicular to the axis of the target coronary vessel (crossed side-to-side anastomosis) (**Figure 15**)

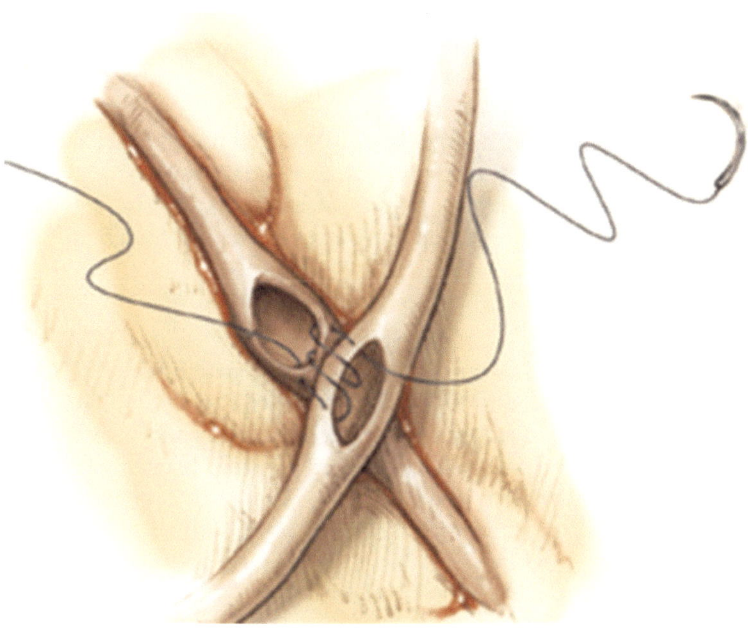

Figure 15.
Crossed side-to-side anastomosis.

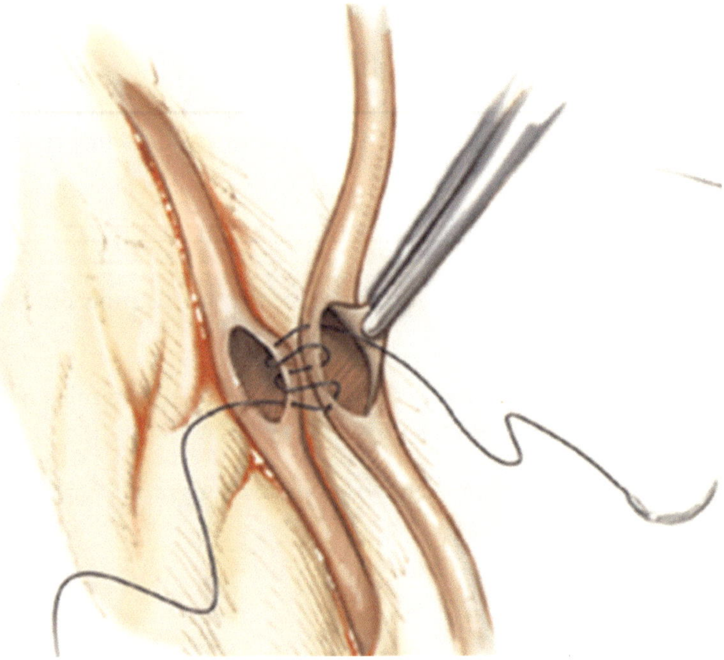

Figure 16.
Parallel side-to-side anastomosis.

2. A parallel configuration in which the graft and target coronary axes are aligned (parallel side-to-side anastomosis) (**Figure 16**)

   - Continuous or interrupted sutures can be used.

   - The side-to-side anastomoses used in SB are technically difficult compared with regular end-to-side anastomoses.

   - Interrupted crossed side-to-side anastomosis greatly simplifies this procedure.

In an experimental study with animals, Shioi [22] compared various techniques for performing anastomoses, reporting that crossed side-to-side anastomosis enabled a larger opening than did parallel side-to-side anastomosis and that interrupted sutures enabled a larger anastomotic opening than did a continuous suture.

6.8 Complications

- **Early death**—in general, after isolated CABG, approximately 98% of patients survive at least 1 month, and 97, 92, 81, and 66% survive 1, 5, 10, and 15 years or more, respectively. In an analysis of seven large datasets representing more than 172,000 patients, Jones and colleagues identified seven variables most predictive of early mortality [23]:

  - Older age

  - Female gender

  - Previous CABG

- Urgency of operation
- Severe LV dysfunction
- Left main disease
- Increased extent of coronary artery disease

- **Adverse neurological outcomes**—a multicenter study by Roach and colleagues of 2108 patients undergoing CABG with CPB documented adverse cerebral outcomes in 129 patients (6.1%) [24]. Type 1 deficits (major focal deficits, stupor, and coma) occurred in 3.1%, and type 2 deficits (deterioration in intellectual function or memory) in 3.0% of the patients. Predictors of type 1 deficits included the presence of proximal aortic arteriosclerosis, history of prior neurologic disease, intra-aortic balloon pump, diabetes, hypertension, unstable angina, and older age.

- **Mediastinitis**—deep sternal wound infection occurs in 1–4% of patients after CABG with CPB and is associated with increased mortality [25]. Obesity is a risk factor for mediastinitis [26]. Other factors associated with an increased prevalence of deep wound infection include diabetes, previous CABG, the use of both IMAs, and duration of operation [26, 27]. Randomized trials have shown that off-pump CABG is not associated with a lower prevalence of sternal wound infection [25, 28].

- **Renal dysfunction**—in a multicenter study of renal dysfunction after CABG with CPB in 2222 patients, “dysfunction” was defined as a postoperative serum creatinine level of 2.0 mg dL^{-1} or greater, or an increase of 0.7 mg dL^{-1} or more from preoperative level [29]. Renal dysfunction occurred in 171 (7.7%) patients, and 30 (1.4%) required dialysis. Early mortality was 0.9% among patients who did not develop renal dysfunction, 19% in those with renal dysfunction who did not require dialysis, and 63% among those who required dialysis. Preoperative risk factors for renal dysfunction included advanced age, moderate to severe cardiac failure, previous CABG, diabetes, and preexisting renal disease [29]. In two randomized trials, prevalence of postoperative renal failure was similar in on-pump and off-pump groups [28, 30].

- **Myocardial infarction**—perioperative MI, usually defined by the appearance of new Q waves in the ECG or non-Q wave MI can also occur which are detected by elevation of serum myocardial biomarkers, is most often related to inappropriate myocardial management, technical problems, or incomplete revascularization. Prevalence of MI is approximately 2.5–5% [31]. Perioperative infarction, when quantitatively more than trivial, is a risk factor for later death [32]. Including perioperative cases, MI is relatively uncommon after CABG, with 94% of patients in the Katholieke Universiteit, Leuven, Belgium (KU Leuven) experience free of infarction for at least 5 years and 73% for at least 15 years [33].

7. Results

- **Unsatisfactory quality of life**—even though unsatisfactory quality of life after CABG is one of the most important unfavorable outcome events, quantifying it is very difficult because it depends on the following three factors:

1. Freedom from angina or heart failure;

2. Freedom from the need for medication, rehospitalization, and reintervention.

3. Preservation of exercise capacity.

Most of the patients have a satisfactory quality of life early after CABG, but this gradually begins to decline after about 5 years [34].

- **Neurobehavioral outcomes**—damaging effects of CPB machine are usually blamed for neurobehavioral disturbances and decline in cognitive function in some patients. These are mild most of the times and might not be apparent unless patients are tested specifically for them. As many as 75% of patients may exhibit these subtle defects when tested 8 days after CABG, but by 3–6 months postoperatively, proportion drops to only about 10–30% [35]. Gross defects most likely result from embolization of arteriosclerotic debris from the ascending aorta or from air and intracardiac thrombus rather than from damaging effects of CPB [36]. Prevalence is about 0.5% in relatively young patients but rises to about 5% in patients older than age 70 and about 8% in those older than 75 [37]. Randomized trials comparing on- and off-pump procedures showed similar prevalence of adverse neurologic outcomes [28].

- **Functional capacity**—maximal exercise capacity of patients is improved by CABG. The degree of exercise capacity depends on preoperative LV function, graft patency, and completeness of revascularization. Maximal exercise capacity generally is improved more by CABG than by medical treatment, at least for 3–10 years [38].

- **Left ventricular function**—resting regional perfusion defects are improved after CABG in at least 65% of patients [39]. Left ventricular wall segments that are hypokinetic, akinetic, or even dyskinetic at rest preoperatively often have improved systolic function after CABG [40]. This is associated with increased regional myocardial perfusion. Improvement in segmental wall motion 12 months after CABG has been observed even in areas of scarring from previous MI [41]. This finding supports the concept that viable muscle cells, which may be hibernating, are scattered through hypokinetic and, at times, even akinetic and dyskinetic segments and that wall motion in such segments can be improved by CABG [42]. When segmental wall contraction does not occur after CABG, incomplete revascularization is the cause in some patients. LV diastolic function, more specifically LV "relaxation," is also improved by successful CABG, and improvement may be immediate [43].

- **Exercise**—the decrease in EF with exercise that is a characteristic of ischemic heart disease is absent 2 weeks after operation in most patients. This favorable response to stress can be brought about only by CABG or PCI and does not result from collateral circulation alone, even when extensive [44]. When global and segmental function during exercise is not improved early (3 months) after operation, one or more bypass grafts are usually occluded or stenosed.

- **Patency of grafts: internal mammary artery**—the highest patency rates for coronary bypass grafts are associated with the use of the left internal mammary (thoracic) artery to bypass the left anterior descending coronary artery. These patency rates are approximately 95% at 10 years after operation, and closure of the mammary artery after that time is uncommon. This favorable performance of the internal mammary artery when anastomosed to the left anterior descending coronary artery is probably due to its particular wall structure and function and the potentially large runoff through the left anterior descending artery system. Internal mammary artery grafts to other vessels appear to have lower patency rates late postoperatively than do those to the left anterior descending artery, and these may be no greater than those of vein grafts [45]. IMA as a free graft from the aorta to LAD provides patency almost as high as with an in situ graft.

- **Other arterial grafts**—early (<13 months) patency of radial artery grafts exceeds 90% and does not differ from ITA patency [46]. A native coronary stenosis of less than 70% is associated with lower patency of a radial artery graft than if the stenosis is 70% or greater. Tatoulis and colleagues [47], in a study of long-term patency of 1108 radial artery grafts, reported patency of 89% at a mean follow-up interval of 48 months. Of 318 grafts in place for more than 5 years, 294 (92%) were patent. Of 107 in place for more than 7 years, 99 (92%) were patent. Patency was highest for grafts placed to the LAD (96%) and lowest for grafts to the RCA (83%).

In a study by Suma and colleagues [48] of gastroepiploic artery grafts in 685 patients who underwent postoperative angiographic evaluation, patency was 91% within 1 year in all 685 patients, 88% between 1 and 5 years in 102 patients and 83% between 5 and 10 years in 102 patients. Time-related patency at 1 month, 1 year, 5 years, and 10 years was 96, 91, 80, and 62%, respectively. The principal causes of late occlusion were anastomotic stenoses and anastomoses to less critically stenosed coronary arteries.

For the inferior epigastric artery, Gurne and colleagues [49] performed postoperative angiography in 122 patients early (11 ± 5 days) and in 72 patients late (11 ± 6 months) after operation. Early patency was 98%, and late patency was 93%. Of 14 grafts that were occluded or threadlike at the late study, 8 were anastomosed to arteries with a stenosis of 60% or less.

- **Saphenous vein grafts**—diffuse intimal hyperplasia is a universal finding in vein grafts that have been in place for more than 1 month [50]. Thickness of the intimal hyperplasia seems to be inversely related to flow in the graft, and the process appears to result in a matching of vein lumen size to that of the coronary arteries supplied by the graft. About 10% of vein grafts get closed within the first few postoperative weeks. By 10 years after insertion, half of vein grafts still patent have undergone at least some arteriosclerotic changes [51]. About 20% of vein grafts have proximal suture line stenosis within 1 year; about one fourth of these are found to be occluded 5 years later. Almost 50% of patients have some narrowing of the distal anastomosis within 1 year, but most have not progressed by 5 years after CABG. The 10-year patency rate of vein grafts appears to be highly variable, and in some reports [52] only 50–60% overall are still patent. Arm veins have a still lower prevalence of patency [53] as do synthetic conduits. The patency rates are lower when the anastomosis is to small coronary arteries and to arteries supplying areas with considerable scar. Thrombosis, another process that can reduce graft patency, may develop early postoperatively. Endothelial cell loss and exposure of the basement membrane and collagen to blood tend to appear early after inserting the vein graft, predisposing it to early accumulation of platelets, fibrin, and thrombus on its luminal surface.

Author details

Mohd. Shahbaaz Khan
King Fahad Medical City, Riyadh, Kingdom of Saudi Arabia

*Address all correspondence to: mohdshahbaazkhan@yahoo.com

References

[1] Benjamin EJ, Blaha MJ, Chiuve SE, et al. Heart disease and stroke Statistics-2017 update: A report from the American Heart Association. Circulation. 2017;**e146**:135

[2] Ganz P, Ganz W. Coronary blood flow and myocardial ischemia. In: Braunwald E, Zipes DP, Libby P, editors. Heart Disease. Philadelphia: W.B. Saunders Company; 2001. pp. 1087-1113

[3] Brandt PW, Partridge JB, Wattie WJ. Coronary angiography: A method of presentation of arteriogram report and a scoring system. Clinical Radiology. 1977; **28**:36

[4] Asirvatham S, Sebastian C, Thadani U. Choosing the most appropriate treatment for stable angina: Safety considerations. Drug Safety. 1998;**19**:23-44

[5] Thadani U. Current medical management of chronic stable angina. Journal of Cardiovascular Pharmacology and Therapeutics. 2004;**9**:S11-S29

[6] Food and Drug Administration. Acetylsalicylic acid and the heart. Journal of the American Medical Association. 1993;**270**:2669

[7] Bhatt DL, Fox KA, Hacke W, et al. Clopidogrel and aspirin versus aspirin alone for the prevention of atherothrombotic events. The New England Journal of Medicine. 2006;**354**: 1706-1717

[8] Pfeffer MA, Braunwald E, Moye LA, et al. Effect of captopril on mortality and morbidity in patients with left ventricular dysfunction after myocardial infarction. The New England Journal of Medicine. 1992;**527**: 669-677

[9] Cooley DA. In memoriam. Tribute to Rene Favaloro, pioneer of coronary bypass. Texas Heart Institute Journal. 2000;**27**:231-232

[10] Vineberg A, Miller G. Internal mammary coronary anastomosis in the surgical treatment of coronary artery insufficiency. Canadian Medical Association Journal. 1951;**64**:204-210

[11] Effler DB. Chapter 1: History. In: Green GE, Singh RN, Sosa JA, editors. Surgical Revascularization of the Heart: The Internal Thoracic Arteries. Tokyo: Igaku-Shoin; 1991. pp. 1-17

[12] Wijnberg DS, Boeve WJ, Ebels T, van Gelder IC, van den Toren EW, Lie KI, et al. Patency of arm vein grafts used in aorto-coronary bypass surgery. European Journal of Cardio-thoracic Surgery. 1990;**4**:510

[13] Culliford AT, Colvin SB, Rohrer K, Baumann G, Spencer FC. The atherosclerotic ascending aorta and transverse arch: A new technique to prevent cerebral injury during bypass: Experience with 13 patients. Annals of Thoracic Surgery. 1986;**41**:27

[14] Aranki SF, Rizzo RJ, Adams DH, Couper GS, Kinchla NM, Gildea JS, et al. Single clamp technique: An important adjunct to myocardial and cerebral protection in coronary operations. The Annals of Thoracic Surgery. 1994;**58**:296

[15] Puskas JD, Thourani VH, Kilgo P, Cooper W, Vassiliades T, Vega JD, et al. Off-pump coronary artery bypass disproportionately benefits high-risk patients. The Annals of Thoracic Surgery. 2009;**88**:1142-1147

[16] Moller CH, Perko MJ, Lund JT, Andersen LW, Kelbaek H, Madsen JK, et al. Three-year follow-up in a subset of high-risk patients randomly assigned to

off-pump versus on-pump coronary artery bypass surgery: The Best Bypass Surgery trial. Heart. 2011;**97**:907-913

[17] Ricci M, Karamanoukian HL, D'Ancona G, Bergsland J, Salerno TA. Exposure and mechanical stabilization in off-pump coronary artery bypass grafting via sternotomy. The Annals of Thoracic Surgery. 2000;**70**:1736

[18] Bergsland J, Karamanoukian HL, Soltoski PR, Salerno TA. "Singlesuture" for circumflex exposure in off-pump coronary artery bypass grafting. The Annals of Thoracic Surgery. 1999;**68**: 1428-1430

[19] Farkouh ME, Domanski M, Sleeper LA, et al. Strategies for multivessel revascularization in patients with diabetes. The New England Journal of Medicine. 2012;**367**:2375-2384

[20] Li J, Liu Y, Zheng J, et al. The patency of sequential and individual vein coronary bypass grafts: A systematic review. The Annals of Thoracic Surgery. 2011;**92**:1292-1298

[21] Schwann TA, Zacharias A, Riordan CJ, Durham SJ, Shah AS, Habib RH. Sequential radial artery grafts for multivessel coronary artery bypass graft surgery: 10-year survival and angiography results. The Annals of Thoracic Surgery. 2009;**88**:31-39

[22] Shioi K. A study of sequential anastomoses in aortocoronary bypass surgery; internal configurations by the casting injection technique. Nagoya Journal of Medical Science. 1984;**46**: 19-26

[23] Jones RH, Hannan EL, Hammermeister KE, Delong ER, O'Connor GT, Luepker RV, et al. Identification of preoperative variables needed for risk adjustment of short-term mortality after coronary artery bypass graft surgery. The Working Group Panel on the Cooperative CABG Database Project. Journal of the American College of Cardiology. 1996;**28**:1478

[24] Roach GW, Kanchuger M, Mangano CM, Newman M, Nussmeier N, Wolman R, et al. Adverse cerebral outcomes after coronary bypass surgery. Multicenter Study of Perioperative Ischemia Research Group and the Ischemia Research and Education Foundation Investigators. The New England Journal of Medicine. 1996;**335**:1857

[25] Shroyer AL, Grover FL, Hattler B, Collins JF, McDonald GO, Kozora E, et al. On-pump versus off-pump coronary-artery bypass surgery. The New England Journal of Medicine. 2009;**361**:1827-1837

[26] Nagachinta T, Stephens M, Reitz B, Polk BF. Risk factors for surgical-wound infection following cardiac surgery. The Journal of Infectious Diseases. 1987;**156**: 967

[27] Kouchoukos NT, Wareing TH, Murphy SF, Pelate C, Marshall WG Jr. Risks of bilateral internal mammary artery bypass grafting. The Annals of Thoracic Surgery. 1990;**49**:210

[28] Bull DA, Neumayer LA, Stringham JC, Meldrum P, Affleck DG, Karwande SV. Coronary artery bypass grafting with cardiopulmonary bypass versus off-pump cardiopulmonary bypass grafting: Does eliminating the pump reduce morbidity and cost? The Annals of Thoracic Surgery. 2001;**71**:170

[29] Mangano CM, Diamondstone LS, Ramsay JG, Aggarwal A, Herskowitz A, Mangano DT. Renal dysfunction after myocardial revascularization: Risk factors, adverse outcomes, and hospital resource utilization. Annals of Internal Medicine. 1998;**128**:194

[30] van Dijk D, Nierich AP, Jansen EW, Nathoe HM, Suyker WJ, Diephuis JC,

et al. Early outcome after off-pump versus on-pump coronary bypass surgery: Results from a randomized study. Circulation. 2001;**104**:1761

[31] Klatte K, Chaitman BR, Theroux P, Gavard JA, Stocke K, Boyce S, et al. Increased mortality after coronary artery bypass graft surgery is associated with increased levels of postoperative creatine kinase-myocardial band isoenzyme release: Results from GUARDIAN trial. Journal of the American College of Cardiology. 2001;**38**:1070

[32] Schaff HV, Gersh BJ, Fisher LD, Frye RL, Mock MB, Ryan TJ, et al. Detrimental effect of perioperative myocardial infarction on late survival after coronary artery bypass. Report from the Coronary Artery Surgery Study—CASS. The Journal of Thoracic and Cardiovascular Surgery. 1984;**88**:972

[33] Sergeant PT, Blackstone EH, Meyns BP. Does arterial revascularization decrease the risk of infarction after coronary artery bypass grafting? The Annals of Thoracic Surgery. 1998;**66**:1

[34] Booth DC, Deupree RH, Hultgren HN, DeMaria AN, Scott SM, Luchi RJ. Quality of life after bypass surgery for unstable angina. 5-year follow-up results of a Veterans Affairs Cooperative Study. Circulation. 1991; **83**:87

[35] Newman MF, Kirchner JL, Phillips-Bute B, Gaver V, Grocott H, Jones RH, et al. Longitudinal assessment of neurocognitive function after coronary-artery bypass surgery. The New England Journal of Medicine. 2001;**344**:395

[36] Katz ES, Tunick PA, Rusinek H, Ribakove G, Spencer FC, Kronzon I. Protruding aortic atheromas predict stroke in elderly patients undergoing cardiopulmonary bypass: Experience with intraoperative transesophageal echocardiography. Journal of the American College of Cardiology. 1992; **20**:70

[37] Tarakji KG, Sabik JF 3rd, Bhudia SK, Batizy LH, Blackstone EH. Temporal onset, risk factors, and outcomes associated with stroke after coronary artery bypass grafting. JAMA. 2011;**305**: 381-390

[38] Mathur VS, Guinn GA. Prospective randomized study to evaluate coronary bypass surgery: 10 year follow-up. Circulation. 1982;**66**:II219

[39] Rubenson DS, Tucker CR, London E, Miller DC, Stinson EB, Popp RL. Two-dimensional echocardiographic analysis of segmental left ventricular wall motion before and after coronary artery bypass surgery. Circulation. 1982;**66**:1025

[40] Lazar HL, Plehn JF, Schick EM, Dobnick D, Shemin RJ. Effects of coronary revascularization on regional wall motion. The Journal of Thoracic and Cardiovascular Surgery. 1989;**98**:498

[41] Mintz LJ, Ingels NB Jr, Daughters GT 2nd, Stinson EB, Alderman EL. Sequential studies of left ventricular function and wall motion after coronary arterial bypass surgery. The American Journal of Cardiology. 1980;**45**:210

[42] Dilsizian V, Bonow RO, Cannon RO, Tracy CM, Vitale DF, McIntosh CL, et al. The effect of coronary bypass grafting on left ventricular systolic function at rest: Evidence for preoperative subclinical myocardial ischemia. The American Journal of Cardiology. 1988;**61**:1248

[43] Humphrey LS, Topol EJ, Rosenfeld GI, Borkon AM, Baumgartner WA, Gardner TJ, et al. Immediate enhancement of left ventricular relaxation by coronary artery bypass grafting: Intraoperative assessment. Circulation. 1988;**77**:886

[44] Sesto M, Schwarz F. Regional myocardial function at rest and after rapid ventricular pacing in patients after myocardial revascularization by coronary bypass graft or by collateral vessels. The American Journal of Cardiology. 1979;**43**:920

[45] Huddleston CB, Stoney WS, Alford WC, et al. Internal mammary artery grafts: Technical factors influencing patency. The Annals of Thoracic Surgery. 1986;**42**:543-549

[46] Weinschelbaum EE, Macchia A, Caramutti VM, Machain HA, Raffaelli HA, Favaloro MR, et al. Myocardial revascularization with radial and mammary arteries: Initial and mid-term results. The Annals of Thoracic Surgery. 2000;**70**:1378

[47] Tatoulis J, Buxton BF, Fuller JA, Meswani M, Theodore S, Powar N, et al. Long-term patency of 1108 radial arterial-coronary angiograms over 10 years. The Annals of Thoracic Surgery. 2009;**88**:23-30

[48] Suma H, Isomura T, Horii T, Sato T. Late angiographic result of using the right gastroepiploic artery as a graft. The Journal of Thoracic and Cardiovascular Surgery. 2000;**120**:496

[49] Gurne O, Buche M, Chenu P, Paquay JL, Pelgrim JP, Louagie Y, et al. Quantitative angiographic follow-up study of the free inferior epigastric coronary bypass graft. Circulation. 1994;**90**:II148

[50] Smith SH, Geer JC. Morphology of saphenous vein–coronary artery bypass grafts: Seven to 116 months after surgery. Archives of Pathology & Laboratory Medicine. 1983;**107**:13-18

[51] Campeau L, Enjalbert M, Lesperance J, et al. The relation of risk factors to the development of atherosclerosis in saphenous-vein bypass grafts and the progression of disease in the native circulation. The New England Journal of Medicine. 1984; **311**:1329-1332

[52] Bourassa MG, Fisher LD, Campeau L, Gillespie MJ, McConney M, Lesperance J. Long-term fate of bypass grafts: The Coronary Artery Surgery Study (CASS) and Montreal Heart Institute experiences. Circulation. 1985; **72**:V71-V78

[53] Stoney WS, Alford WC, Burrus GR, Glassford DM Jr, Petracek MR, Thomas CS. The fate of arm veins used for aorta-coronary bypass grafts. The Journal of Thoracic and Cardiovascular Surgery. 1984;**88**:522-526

Chapter 6

Early and Late Survival and Associated Factors in Patients Undergoing Coronary Artery Bypass Grafting

Ahmad Amouzeshi and Zahra Amouzeshi

Abstract

Several studies have aimed to compare the early and late survival rates and the related factors in patients who undergo coronary artery bypass grafting (CABG). Among such factors are age, gender, arrhythmia, stroke, serum procalcitonin level, number and type of grafts, diabetes mellitus, chronic kidney disease, chronic obstructive pulmonary disease (COPD), addiction, ejection fraction, transfusion of blood products, and the kind of technique (off-pump versus on-pump). Controversies surround early and late survival and some of the associated factors in patients undergoing CABG. Therefore, it appears vital to compare the early and late survival chances and the related factors after CABG.

Keywords: coronary artery bypass grafting, survival, patients, cardiac surgery

1. Introduction

CABG continues to be the most common procedure in adult cardiac surgery for coronary artery disease [1]. CABG improves survival, particularly in complex diabetic patients, those above 65 years of age, patients with left main stem or triple-vessel disease, and those who have an impairment in the left ventricular function [2].

Many studies have attempted to compare the early and late survival rates and the relevant factors in patients who undergo CABG. A 20-year follow-up investigation of patients undergoing CABG reported lower survival rates as related to the female gender, age, hypertension, previous CABG, angina class, number of vessels diseased, heavyweight, and ejection fraction (EF) [3]. Another study shows that late survival is associated with increased weight, history of myocardial infarction, smoking, diabetes, and application of vein grafts merely in CABG patients [4].

In light of the current controversy over early and late survival rates and some of the related factors in patients undergoing CABG, it seems critically important to compare the early and late survival chances and associated factors after CABG.

1.1 Gender

Most studies report that women hold a higher risk for morbidity and mortality after CABG procedures than their male counterparts do [5, 6]. Abramov's study demonstrated that there is a greater prevalence of most risk factors in women (including old age, urgent operation, prior PTCA, Canadian Cardiovascular Society angina class 3–4, congestive heart failure, hypertension, diabetes mellitus, peripheral vascular disease, and smaller body surface area). Men have a higher prevalence of left ventricular EF of <35%, triple-vessel disease, and history of smoking. Moreover, Abramov's study found that internal mammary artery grafts and multiple arterial grafts were not used as frequently in women as in men [5]. It should be highlighted that a critical difference between men and women is the later onset of coronary artery disease in women. By inference, after age is controlled, female patients undergoing surgery may have a shorter duration of coronary artery disease, which would be associated with longer life [5].

1.2 Age

Demographic changes over the last decades have resulted in a different patient population for surgeons, including cardiac surgeons. It is now typical of elderly patients to have several, relatively severe comorbidities such as hypertension, pulmonary diseases, diabetes, obesity, renal insufficiency, as well as peripheral arterial disease (PAD) [7].

Alongside this, Naughton compared the early and late predictors of mortality after on-pump CABG in an elderly and a younger population, showing that mortality in elderly patients improved substantially, although it remained more than twice that of younger patients. The difference in contributors to early and 1-year mortality implies the need for effectual short- and long-term strategies, especially in controlling chronic diseases such as heart and renal failure [8].

Coronary artery revascularization via CABG surgery or percutaneous coronary intervention in 80-year-old patients or older can have satisfactory in-hospital and 2-year clinical outcomes. Nevertheless, recovery may be prolonged in up to 20% of patients, and they may not be immediately able to leave the hospital [9].

In Nicolini's study [10], patients younger than 60 years undergoing CABG showed a lower risk of undesirable outcomes than older patients. Patients younger than 60 have a different clinical pattern of coronary artery disease (CAD) presentation as compared to more elderly patients. Especially speaking, the factors of obesity, male gender, the history of myocardial infarction, the history of PCI, and the presence of depressed left ventricular function, have been found to be highly commonplace among patients younger than 60. Focused attention should be directed to these issues if one aims to design and improve preventive strategies than can alleviate the effect of specific cardiovascular risk factors for younger patients, including lifestyle, diet, and weight control. More research with longer follow-up periods should be performed to investigate the efficacy and durability of myocardial revascularization in younger patients in need of CABG [10].

1.3 Biomarkers

According to Petäjä's meta-analysis, postoperative CK-MB release is linked with survival up to 40 months after surgery. Troponin levels can assumedly be better predictors of mortality than CK-MB due to their specificity to the myocardium [11].

Also, high levels of postoperative serum procalcitonin have been demonstrated to correlate with infection, mortality, and other severe post-cardiac surgery complications [12]. Dörge et al. revealed that survival rates in the first 24 h after the operation are lower in patients with high levels of serum PCT [13]. Fritz et al. [14] also reported that a PCT level greater than 2.5 ng l^{-1} could be predictive of mortality within the first 28 days after CABG surgery [14].

1.4 Type of grafts

Completeness of revascularization is contingent upon the number of grafts required, the type of graft, and the number of grafts performed [15]. Saphenous vein grafts (SVG) are the most frequently employed conduits from among arterial and venous conduits for CABG surgery. It is because they are characterized by superficial access site and reduced risk for bleeding compared with arterial conduits. Endoscopic SVG harvest was reported to have short-term graft patency similar to open SVG harvest, although there are concerns for a significantly reduced long-term graft patency at 12 months and beyond. Given the potential implications of endoscopic SVG harvest for deteriorated long-term outcomes in patients undergoing CABG, its role has received much controversy in the literature, although it is generally considered non-subsidiary to open harvest [1].

Amouzeshi's study showed that EVH is a safe and minimally invasive technique for vein harvesting and that it can decrease the harvest time and postoperative pain. Moreover, the efficiency of EVH and OVH is similar. Nevertheless, further research is needed to probe into its cosmetic outcomes, cost-efficiency, and hospital costs; it is even more essential to study the long-term graft patency of the EVH technique [16].

The systematic review and meta-analysis conducted by Kodia on 18,131 patients undergoing CABG showed greater patency via open SVG harvest than endoscopic SVG harvest after a follow-up of around 2.5 years. Patients with open SVG harvest showed higher rates of early wound complications and postoperative 30-day mortality, which, importantly, did not mean differences in overall mortality [1].

Finally, Grau's study indicated that bilateral internal mammary artery had better outcomes than single internal mammary artery [17].

A meta-analysis incorporating 27 studies and over 79,000 patients revealed a higher survival rate among patients who received bilateral internal mammary artery (BIMA) as compared with those who underwent left internal mammary artery for CABG surgery. While it is imperative to tailor the surgery to each patient, no one can disregard the advantage and gain from this operative strategy. Moreover, given the reduced rates of short-term morbidity (i.e., deep sternal wound infection) through better operative techniques, BIMA bypass grafting can be a first-line alternative for patients receiving revascularization [18].

1.5 Stroke

Stroke is a primary cause of morbidity and mortality following CABG. It continues to be one of the most disabling and damaging complications of CABG, which carries significant clinical and economic implications for both patients and the healthcare system [19, 20]. Moreover, it is a potentially preventable complication of CABG [20].

The results from Tarakji's study on patients undergoing CABG at a single center during a 30-year period showed that the incidence of stroke reduced despite an increasing patient risk profile and that over half of strokes occurred postoperatively rather than intraoperatively. Clinical presentation and surgical technique were specific to intraoperative stroke, but age and arteriosclerotic burden were associated with both intraoperative and postoperative strokes [20].

In Mao's study, seven variables (including advanced age, prior carotid artery stenosis, history of cerebrovascular disease/stroke, prior peripheral vascular disease, prior unstable angina, prolonged cardiopulmonary bypass time, and postoperative atrial fibrillation), representing high atherosclerotic burden, were found related to perioperative stroke events [19].

In the course of a surgical procedure, there are three different mechanisms that may trigger postoperative strokes: (1) embolic events, (2) defects in brain perfusion, and (3) an inflammatory response, which can, in cases, intensify the other mechanisms [21].

Postoperative neurological complications, particularly those with a deficit, are especially destructive. Mainly, they are the outcome of macroparticle emboli associated with aortic atherosclerosis. It stands as a paradox that off-pump surgery has provided for a better recognition of the numerous pathophysiological processes, which might induce postoperative complications, most notably the neurological difficulties. It is now possible to measure the benefits that have become available by modified surgical practices and cardiopulmonary bypass (CPB). Modification of current cardiological therapies, with an increased use of antiplatelet agents and preoperative interventional procedures, may alter the surgical scene. As a result, many pathophysiological aspects may need further research [21].

1.6 Arrhythmia

Atrial fibrillation (AF) is one of the most common complications following cardiac surgery. It may happen in ~20–35% of cases after CABG surgery and in over 50% of patients upon valve surgery. AF after cardiac surgery is a primary cause of morbidity and mortality in patients [22].

In case preoperative atrial fibrillation is left uncorrected in patients undergoing CABG, it has been demonstrated that greater late cardiac morbidity and mortality as well as poorer long-term survival will follow. Thus, atrial fibrillation surgery should be considered at the time of CABG. It has yet to be determined whether the ablation of atrial fibrillation at the time of CABG can enhance prognosis, yet the present data support the idea of considering concurrent AF surgery [23].

Also, prior AF in patients who undergo CABG has been recognized as an incremental risk factor for time-related mortality. Even after being adjusted for risk factors of stroke, the patients with AF have a more substantial stroke risk of 2.6–4.5 times. The reason for the late increased mortality in patients with AF is not well known. Unquestionably, the higher chance of stroke and bleeding is explained by some of the difference; however, several studies also indicate that chronic tachycardia is linked with late mortality [24].

1.7 Diabetes mellitus (DM)

Patients suffering from DM bear a higher chance of adverse outcomes after CABG [25]. Thourani's study showed that DM has both worse in-hospital and long-term outcomes after CABG. The increased risk in DM patients can only partially be accounted for by demographic characteristics. Moreover, this study showed that diabetic patients were older and had more extensive coronary artery disease, a lower preoperative EF, a higher incidence of hypertension, prior myocardial infarction, heart failure, and class III–IV angina at the time of presentation [26].

In Zoltan Szabo's study, diabetic patients could undergo CABG in case they had an acceptable mortality risk, which was only slightly different from that found in nondiabetic patients. Cardiac grounds for early mortality were predominant in both diabetic and nondiabetic patients. However, the neurologic injury was evidence for a relatively higher proportion of early deaths in diabetic patients. Besides, midterm survival was noticeably compromised, especially in diabetic patients treated with insulin [27].

Calafiore's study showed that diabetes is an independent risk factor only for early cardiac mortality. Long-term survival in those who live the first 30 days does not differ significantly in diabetic and nondiabetic patients. In fact, the rates are very close [28].

A large 11-year-long nationwide cohort of patients undergoing a first isolated CABG in Sweden showed that the risk of death after CABG was double in patients with type 1 DM (T1DM) than patients without DM. Moreover, the cohort found that patients with type 2 diabetes mellitus (T2DM) had almost a similar risk of death as patients without diabetes. According to the cohort, patients with T1DM grow a high risk of adverse outcomes after CABG and should be intently followed up. Moreover, all possible measures need to be taken to reduce the risks of mortality or recurrent cardiovascular events in them [25].

Therefore, diabetic patients form a significant portion of the population undergoing surgical coronary revascularization.

1.8 Chronic kidney disease (CKD)

Creatinine levels are of a crucial role in on-pump coronary bypass grafting mortality. A worse prognosis may result from the combination of some risk factors and higher admission creatinine values. Moreover, lower admission creatinine values have been linked with a protective impact, even among elderly patients and those with a high cardiopulmonary bypass time [29].

Miceli's study indicates that occult renal dysfunction, i.e., normal creatinine level with impaired renal function, is connected with higher mortality and postoperative morbidity in CABG patients. A precise assessment of renal function, by estimating creatinine clearance and serum creatinine, can help detect patients at higher risks and categorize risks more accurately so that therapeutic strategies can be better optimized for these patients [30].

1.9 Chronic obstructive pulmonary disease (COPD)

Chronic obstructive pulmonary disease is associated with prolonged mechanical ventilation, prolonged length of stay, and postoperative complications such as pneumonia. It is similarly a principal predictor of long-term survival after CABG [31].

In one meta-analysis study (2019), COPD was not predictive of increased risks of postoperative mortality after CABG. Nevertheless, the study revealed that patients with COPD developed higher chances of developing postoperative morbidities, especially pneumonia, respiratory failure, renal failure, stroke, and wound infection. Therefore, when a patient with COPD requires CABG, caution should be taken in light of the higher risk for developing postoperative complications as with the respiratory system and others. High-quality RCTs are needed to confirm these results, however [32].

In Efird's study [31], COPD and prolonged length of stay were two of the several contributors to long-term postoperative mortality in CABG patients. In this regard, to reduce length of stay after CABG, it might be necessary to take aggressive treatment strategies with an aim for early weaning off of mechanical ventilation and prevention of reintubation among COPD patients. Our findings also have important implications for the long-term management of these patients and strategies for managing costs as the patient lives on [31].

1.10 Type of technique (off-pump versus on-pump)

Many studies have investigated the outcomes of off-pump and on-pump CABG. Nevertheless, their results are contradictory, and the advantages and disadvantages of the two methods are not clearly explained [33, 34]. Some studies have argued for the superior outcomes of off-pump CABG, primarily as concerned with short- and long-term mortality rates and complications. However, some other studies have reported no significant differences between the two techniques [35, 36]. As an example, in a meta-analysis of mid- and long-term outcomes (2014), off-pump and on-pump CABG conferred similar midterm survival rates. On-pump CABG, however, was connected with better chances of long-term survival [36].

According to the results of Amouzeshi's study, the outcomes (e.g., death, myocardial infarction, rehospitalization, and normal physical activity) were not significantly different between off-pump and on-pump CABG in patients who underwent primary isolated non-emergent CABG during a 6-year follow-up phase [15].

In Raja's study, off-pump CABG versus on-pump CABG is correlated with comparable short-, mid-, and long-term mortality, similar organ protection, and fewer distal anastomoses. The available evidence cannot, nonetheless, substantiate all concerns about the safety and efficacy of off-pump CABG [37].

1.11 Addiction

Opioids are generally used as anesthetic agents. Long-term application of opioids can lead to analgesic tolerance via an unclear mechanism. Thus, addicted patients may require higher opioid doses [38].

Opiate addiction in CABG patients is of relatively high prevalence. Some studies indicate that drug addiction increases postoperative bleeding and risks of readmission in patients undergoing CABG. Besides, drug addiction together with pain suppression and changes in the endocrine system and cytokines can alter the process of wound healing in patients undergoing surgery [39].

Nemati's study showed that inhalational opium addiction is linked with higher bleeding after CABG. Given the overwhelming number of individuals with opium addiction who might need CABG in countries where opium addiction is widespread, cardiac surgeons need to consider these patients as being at high risk for major complications after surgery [40].

Given the fairly high prevalence of opium abuse among patients undergoing cardiac surgery and its potential prediction of AF after cardiac surgery, cardiac surgeons need to take better preventive measures when planning surgery for opium addict patients [22].

1.12 Ejection fraction

In patients undergoing CABG, the grade of left ventricular EF impairment, which reflects a decreased amount of contracting myocardium, stands as a recognized risk factor for poor short-term and long-term prognoses [41].

Patients with low EF are at higher risks of ventricular arrhythmia, sudden death, and deteriorating heart failure because of recurrent ischemia. In patients with low EF, CABG is demonstrated to be superior to medical therapy alone, leading to significant clinical enhancement and improved long-term survival [42].

Pieri's study [43] showed that moderate-to-severe left ventricular dysfunction is a typical finding in the general population undergoing cardiac surgery. Those with reduced low preoperative left ventricular EF undergoing cardiac surgery carry a high risk of postoperative complications as well as a higher mortality rate. However, the operation can be performed with a comparatively low mortality rate [43].

Haxhibeqiri-Karabdic's study [44] showed that in patients with left ventricular dysfunction, CABG could be performed safely with improvement in life quality and left ventricular EF.

Developments in preoperative management, enhancements in surgical techniques, application of off-pump CABG, advances in cardiac anesthesia, and improvement in intensive postoperative care have led to a decreased mortality rate in patients with low EF operated by off-pump CABG [42].

Inamdar's study [42] revealed that in patients with coronary artery disease and low EF, off-pump CABG could be performed as a relatively safe procedure. It results in good midterm survival, improved left ventricular function, and enhanced overall life quality [42].

Amouzeshi's study [45] showed that even though an EF below 30% is an independent risk factor of mortality, proper care could minimize mortality after CABG. Besides, the study suggested inquiring into the impact of length of time after surgery and variables such as postoperative hospital care, surgical technique, the surgeon himself, and patient self-care training in more hospitals. It is necessary to note that the mortality rate of 10% in patients with EF below 30 and 5% in patients with EF above 30% in this investigation is quite satisfactory according to global standards [34].

Moreover, it is critical to have a careful preoperative selection and operative management, including optimal strategies of myocardial preservation for patients with low EF undergoing cardiac surgery [45].

1.13 Transfusion of blood products

Transfusion of blood products in patients undergoing CABG is linked with higher mortality and morbidity [46]. A few studies have revealed an association between blood transfusion and lower long-term survival after CABG [47].

Van Straten's study revealed that the number of transfused RBC is an independent predictor of early but not late mortality after CABG. Compared to the expected survival, receiving no RBC improves the patient's long-term survival, whereas receiving three or more units of RBC decreases the patient's survival significantly [46].

Mikkola's study showed that transfusion of any blood product is connected with significantly increased risks of all-cause and cardiac mortality after CABG. Such risks seem to be confined to the early postoperative period and decline later on. The perioperative use of fresh frozen plasma or Octaplas, from among blood products, appears to be the primary predictor of mortality [47].

These findings suggest that patient blood management is of extreme importance in enhancing postoperative outcomes, even in low-risk patients undergoing CABG [48].

2. Conclusions

In addition to cardiac-related and operation-related factors, patient-related contributors including senior age, comorbidity, female gender, and clinical preoperative situation can affect the clinical outcome of patients after CABG. This surgical procedure is a multidimensional phenomenon. In this regard, cardiac rehabilitation/secondary prevention programs can play a critical role in enhancing the process of care and outcome of this growing high-risk group of patients.

Acknowledgements

This research did not have any grant from agencies in the public, commercial, or not-for-profit sectors.

Conflict of interest

The authors declare no conflict of interest in this study.

Author details

Ahmad Amouzeshi[1] and Zahra Amouzeshi[2*]

1 Department of Cardiovascular Surgery, Atherosclerosis and Coronary Artery Research Centre, School of Medicine, Birjand University of Medical Sciences, Birjand, Iran

2 Faculty of Nursing and Midwifery, Atherosclerosis and Coronary Artery Research Centre, Birjand University of Medical Sciences, Birjand, Iran

*Address all correspondence to: amouzeshiz9039@gmail.com
and amoozeshiz9039@bums.ac.ir

References

[1] Kodia K, Patel S, Weber MP, Luc JG, Choi JH, Maynes EJ, et al. Graft patency after open versus endoscopic saphenous vein harvest in coronary artery bypass grafting surgery: A systematic review and meta-analysis. Annals of Cardiothoracic Surgery. 2018;**7**(5):586

[2] ElBardissi AW, Aranki SF, Sheng S, O'Brien SM, Greenberg CC, Gammie JS. Trends in isolated coronary artery bypass grafting: An analysis of the society of thoracic surgeons adult cardiac surgery database. The Journal of Thoracic and Cardiovascular Surgery. 2012;**143**(2):273-281

[3] Weintraub WS, Clements SD Jr, Crisco LV-T, Guyton RA, Craver JM, Jones EL, et al. Twenty-year survival after coronary artery surgery: An institutional perspective from Emory University. Circulation. 2003;**107**(9):1271-1277

[4] Myers WO, Blackstone EH, Davis K, Foster ED, Kaiser GC. CASS registry: Long term surgical survival. Journal of the American College of Cardiology. 1999;**33**(2):488-498

[5] Abramov D, Tamariz MG, Sever JY, Christakis GT, Bhatnagar G, Heenan AL, et al. The influence of gender on the outcome of coronary artery bypass surgery. The Annals of Thoracic Surgery. 2000;**70**(3):800-805

[6] Brandrup-Wognsen G, Berggren H, Hartford M, Hjalmarson Å, Karlsson T, Herlitz J. Female sex is associated with increased mortality and morbidity early, but not late, after coronary artery bypass grafting. European Heart Journal. 1996;**17**(9):1426-1431

[7] Kolat P, Ried M, Haneya A, Philipp A, Kobuch R, Hirt S, et al. Impact of age on early outcome after coronary bypass graft surgery using minimized versus conventional extracorporeal circulation. Journal of Cardiothoracic Surgery. 2014;**9**(1):143

[8] Naughton C, Feneck RO, Roxburgh J. Early and late predictors of mortality following on-pump coronary artery bypass graft surgery in the elderly as compared to a younger population. European Journal of Cardio-Thoracic Surgery. 2009;**36**(4):621-627

[9] Garza JJ, Gantt DS, Van Cleave H, Riggs MW, Dehmer GJ. Hospital disposition and long-term follow-up of patients aged ≥ 80 years undergoing coronaryartery revascularization. The American Journal of Cardiology. 2003;**92**(5):590-592

[10] Nicolini F, Fortuna D, Contini GA, Pacini D, Gabbieri D, Zussa C, et al. The impact of age on clinical outcomes of coronary artery bypass grafting: Long-term results of a real-world registry. BioMed Research International. 2017;**2017**:1-11

[11] Petäjä L, Salmenperä M, Pulkki K, Pettilä V. Biochemical injury markers and mortality after coronary artery bypass grafting: A systematic review. The Annals of Thoracic Surgery. 2009;**87**(6):1981-1992.e3

[12] Prat C, Ricart P, Ruyra X, Domínguez J, Morillas J, Blanco S, et al. Serum concentrations of procalcitonin after cardiac surgery. Journal of Cardiac Surgery. 2008;**23**(6):627-632

[13] Dörge H, Schöndube F, Dörge P, Seipelt R, Voss M, Messmer B. Procalcitonin is a valuable prognostic marker in cardiac surgery but not specific for infection. The Thoracic and Cardiovascular Surgeon. 2003;**51**(06):322-326

[14] Fritz H, Brandes H, Bredle D, Bitterlich A, Vollandt R, Specht M, et al. Post-operative hypoalbuminaemia and

procalcitonin elevation for prediction of outcome in cardiopulmonary bypass surgery. Acta Anaesthesiologica Scandinavica. 2003;**47**(10):1276-1283

[15] Amouzeshi A, Amouzeshi Z, Teshnizi MA, Moeinipour AA, Maleki MH. Off-pump versus on-pump coronary artery bypass graft surgery outcomes during 6 years: A prospective cohort study. Acta Medica Iranica. 2017;**55**(9):578-584

[16] Amouzeshi A, Teshnisi MA, Zirak N, Shamloo AS, Hoseinikhah H, Alizadeh B, et al. Clinicopathological comparisons of open vein harvesting and endoscopic vein harvesting in coronary artery bypass grafting patients in Mashhad. Electronic Physician. 2016;**8**(1):1693

[17] Grau JB, Johnson CK, Kuschner CE, Ferrari G, Shaw RE, Brizzio ME, et al. Impact of pump status and conduit choice in coronary artery bypass: A 15-year follow-up study in 1412 propensity-matched patients. The Journal of Thoracic and Cardiovascular Surgery. 2015;**149**(4):1027-1033.e2

[18] Weiss AJ, Zhao S, Tian DH, Taggart DP, Yan TD. A meta-analysis comparing bilateral internal mammary artery with left internal mammary artery for coronary artery bypass grafting. Annals of Cardiothoracic Surgery. 2013;**2**(4):390

[19] Mao Z, Zhong X, Yin J, Zhao Z, Hu X, Hackett ML. Predictors associated with stroke after coronary artery bypass grafting: A systematic review. Journal of the Neurological Sciences. 2015;**357**(1-2):1-7

[20] Tarakji KG, Sabik JF, Bhudia SK, Batizy LH, Blackstone EH. Temporal onset, risk factors, and outcomes associated with stroke after coronary artery bypass grafting. JAMA. 2011;**305**(4):381-390

[21] Baufreton C. Role of surgical factors in strokes after cardiac surgery. Archives of Cardiovascular Diseases. 2010;**103**(5):326-332

[22] Soleimani A, Habibi MR, Hasanzadeh Kiabi F, Emami Zeydi A. Opium addiction as a novel predictor of atrial fibrillation after cardiac surgery. International Cardiovascular Research Journal. 2012;**6**(3):96

[23] Ngaage DL, Schaff HV, Mullany CJ, Sundt IIITM, Dearani JA, Barnes S, et al. Does preoperative atrial fibrillation influence early and late outcomes of coronary artery bypass grafting? The Journal of Thoracic and Cardiovascular Surgery. 2007;**133**(1):182-189

[24] Quader MA, McCarthy PM, Gillinov AM, Alster JM, Cosgrove IIIDM, Lytle BW, et al. Does preoperative atrial fibrillation reduce survival after coronary artery bypass grafting? The Annals of Thoracic Surgery. 2004;**77**(5):1514-1524

[25] Holzmann MJ, Rathsman B, Eliasson B, Kuhl J, Svensson A-M, Nyström T, et al. Long-term prognosis in patients with type 1 and 2 diabetes mellitus after coronary artery bypass grafting. Journal of the American College of Cardiology. 2015;**65**(16):1644-1652

[26] Thourani VH, Weintraub WS, Stein B, Gebhart SS, Craver JM, Jones EL, et al. Influence of diabetes mellitus on early and late outcome after coronary artery bypass grafting. The Annals of Thoracic Surgery. 1999;**67**(4):1045-1052

[27] Szabó Z, Håkanson E, Svedjeholm R. Early postoperative outcome and medium-term survival in 540 diabetic and 2239 nondiabetic patients undergoing coronary artery bypass grafting. The Annals of Thoracic Surgery. 2002;**74**(3):712-719

[28] Calafiore AM, Di Mauro M, Di Giammarco G, Contini M, Vitolla G,

Iacò AL, et al. Effect of diabetes on early and late survival after isolated first coronary bypass surgery in multivessel disease. The Journal of Thoracic and Cardiovascular Surgery. 2003;**125**(1):144-154

[29] Oliveira MA, Santos CA, Brandi AC, Dotta AH, Botelho PH, Godoy MF, et al. Effect of preoperative creatinine levels on mortality after coronary artery bypass grafting surgery: An observational study. Brazilian Journal of Cardiovascular Surgery. 2019;**34**(2):149-155

[30] Miceli A, Bruno VD, Capoun R, Romeo F, Angelini GD, Caputo M. Occult renal dysfunction: A mortality and morbidity risk factor in coronary artery bypass grafting surgery. The Journal of Thoracic and Cardiovascular Surgery. 2011;**141**(3):771-776

[31] Efird JT, Griffin W, O'Neal WT, Davies SW, Shiue KY, Grzybowski M, et al. Long-term survival after cardiac surgery in patients with chronic obstructive pulmonary disease. American Journal of Critical Care. 2016;**25**(3):266-276

[32] Zhao H, Li L, Yang G, Gong J, Ye L, Zhi S, et al. Postoperative outcomes of patients with chronic obstructive pulmonary disease undergoing coronary artery bypass grafting surgery: A meta-analysis. Medicine. 2019;**98**(6):e14388

[33] Bakaeen FG, Chu D, Kelly RF, Holman WL, Jessen ME, Ward HB. Perioperative outcomes after on-and off-pump coronary artery bypass grafting. Texas Heart Institute Journal. 2014;**41**(2):144-151

[34] Dhurandhar V, Saxena A, Parikh R, Vallely MP, Wilson MK, Butcher JK, et al. Outcomes of on-pump versus off-pump coronary artery bypass graft surgery in the high risk (AusSCORE > 5). Heart, Lung & Circulation. 2015;**24**(12):1216-1224

[35] Dalén M, Ivert T, Holzmann MJ, Sartipy U. Long-term survival after off-pump coronary artery bypass surgery: A Swedish nationwide cohort study. The Annals of Thoracic Surgery. 2013;**96**(6):2054-2060

[36] Chaudhry UA, Harling L, Rao C, Ashrafian H, Ibrahim M, Kokotsakis J, et al. Off-pump versus on-pump coronary revascularization: Meta-analysis of mid- and long-term outcomes. The Annals of Thoracic Surgery. 2014;**98**(2):563-572

[37] Raja S. Off-pump versus on-pump coronary artery bypass grafting: Comparative effectiveness. Journal of Comparative Effectiveness Research. 2015;**5**:73-79

[38] Mottahedi B, Ghodsi M, Zargaran B, Hajebi Khaniki S, Komeilipour M, Kahrom M. Consequences of coronary artery bypass grafting in smokers and addicts. Journal of Cardio-Thoracic Medicine. 2018;**6**(3):332-337

[39] Amouzeshi A, Dolatabadi M, Nakhaee S, Maleki MH, Mehrpour O. Comparing short-term mortality in opium users and non-users candidate for coronary artery bypass graft surgery. Journal of Surgery and Trauma. 2017;**5**(1-2):13-17

[40] Nemati MH, Astaneh B, Ardekani GS. Effects of opium addiction on bleeding after coronary artery bypass graft surgery: Report from Iran. General Thoracic and Cardiovascular Surgery. 2010;**58**(9):456-460

[41] Dalén M, Lund LH, Ivert T, Holzmann MJ, Sartipy U. Survival after coronary artery bypass grafting in patients with preoperative heart failure and preserved vs reduced ejection fraction. JAMA Cardiology. 2016;**1**(5):530-538

[42] Inamdar AK, Shende SP, Inamdar SA. Outcome of coronary artery bypass graft surgery in patients

with low ejection fraction. Medical Journal of Dr DY Patil University. 2017;**10**(2):162

[43] Pieri M, Belletti A, Monaco F, Pisano A, Musu M, Dalessandro V, et al. Outcome of cardiac surgery in patients with low preoperative ejection fraction. BMC Anesthesiology. 2016;**16**(1):97

[44] Haxhibeqiri-KarabdicI, HasanovicA, Kabil E, Straus S. Improvement of ejection fraction after coronary artery bypass grafting surgery in patients with impaired left ventricular function. Medical Archives. 2014;**68**(5):332

[45] Amouzeshi A, Zanguoie M, Shakhsemampour B. A survival after coronary artery bypass grafting surgery with ejection fraction below 30 percent. Addiction. 2018;**3**:0.01

[46] Van Straten AH, Bekker MW, Soliman Hamad MA, Van Zundert AA, Martens EJ, Schönberger JP, et al. Transfusion of red blood cells: The impact on short-term and long-term survival after coronary artery bypass grafting, a ten-year follow-up. Interactive Cardiovascular and Thoracic Surgery. 2010;**10**(1):37-42

[47] Mikkola R, Heikkinen J, Lahtinen J, Paone R, Juvonen T, Biancari F. Does blood transfusion affect intermediate survival after coronary artery bypass surgery? Scandinavian Journal of Surgery. 2013;**102**(2):110-116

[48] Kinnunen EM, De Feo M, Reichart D, Tauriainen T, Gatti G, Onorati F, et al. Incidence and prognostic impact of bleeding and transfusion after coronary surgery in low-risk patients. Transfusion. 2017;**57**(1):178-186

Chapter 7

Should We Do Bilateral Internal Mammary Artery Grafting in Diabetic Patients?

Hassane Abdallah, Ahmed Ibrahim and Khalid Al Khamees

Abstract

Nowadays, potential advantages of BIMA grafting are recognized overall in terms of long-term survival1 and by not increasing operative morbidity. One of the major restrictions for extending the use of BIMA grafting is the current impossibility of generalizing the procedure to higher risk patients. These results tend to confirm recent results that promote the use of BIMA grafting in every kind of patients and consequently to confirm the generalization of the procedure, without being afraid of sternal complications. The absence of deep sternal wound infection in our study shows that there is no contraindication of BITA grafting among diabetic patients.

Keywords: coronary, diabetes, deep sternal wound infection

1. Background

Coronary artery disease (CAD) is the most common pathology which prepossesses cardiologists and cardiac surgeons in the past century. Ischemic heart disease was also the most common reason of mortality in the world as reported by the World Health Organization in 2018 [1].

While Coronary artery bypass grafting (CABG) is the preferred therapeutic option for ischemic heart disease in diabetic patients, surgical modalities of the procedure are still debated. One of these is the choice of grafts. Single internal-thoracic-artery graft has resulted in a 10-year rate of angiographic patency exceeding 90%, as compared with 50% for vein grafts. These excellent long-term outcomes have stimulated the use of a bilateral internal-thoracic-artery approach. Nevertheless, the technique is associated to a major drawback. By compromising severely the sternal vascularization, the BIMA may expose patients higher rates of sternal wound infection and this risk seems to be particularly increased in diabetic patients.

The purpose of this chapter is to assess, according to our experience and literature review, the feasibility and the safety of BIMA in patients with diabetes undergoing CABG. Furthermore, the paper highlighted the importance of some cautions and adjunct measures that should be adopted systematically.

2. Patients and methods

A retrospective analysis of the patients who underwent coronary artery bypass surgery in our institution from January 2017 to January 2019 was performed.

All the data were retrieved from computer based medical records. All patients were followed-up in our hospital after the discharge.

The incidence of postoperative sternal wound infections in diabetic patients who received bilateral internal thoracic artery grafting was compared with the incidence

Variable	Total	Diabetic (n = 116)	Non –diabetic (n – 94)	*P* value
Age	**52.1 ± 9**	**52.9 ± 7.9**	**51. 04 ± 10.2**	**0.2**
≤50 year	98(47%)	50(24%)	48(23%)	0.3
>50 year	112(53%)	66(31%)	46(22%)	
Sex				
Female	10(5%)	4(2%)	6(3%)	0.3
Male	200(95%)	112(53%)	88(42%)	
HbAIc(mean ± SD)	**7.8 ± 1.8**	8.8 ± 1.6	6.1 ± 0.7	0.0001
≤7	95(45%)	27(13%)	65(31%)	0.0001
>7	78(37%)	71(34%)	8(4%)	
≥10	37(18%)	39(18%)	0(0%)	
HbAIc > 7 and BMI > 30	**69(33%)**	**63(54%)**	**6(6%)**	**0.0001**
BMI(mean ± SD)	**29.1 ± 4.6**	**29.2 ± 4.7**	**28.7 ± 4.5**	**0.5**
<25	59(28%)	29(14%)	29(14%)	0.3
25–30	76(36%)	46(22%)	29(14%)	
>30–35	52(25%)	32(15%)	21(10%)	
>35–40	23(11%)	13(6%)	11(5%)	
EF				
<30	34(16%)	21(10%)	13(6%)	0.7
30–50	69(33%)	40(19%)	29(14%)	
>50	107(51%)	59(28%)	48(23%)	

Table 1.
Preoperative characteristics (n = 210).

Variable	Diabetic	Non-diabetic	*P* value
Number of coronary by anastomosis (mean)	2.7	2.6	0.4
Y fashion			
No	99(47%)	73(35%)	0.6
Yes	23(11%)	15(7%)	
Pump			
Off	72(35%)	60(29%)	0.7
On	44(21%)	34(16%)	
Cross clamp time in minutes (Mean ± SD)	37 ± 6	41 ± 7	0.002
Bypass surgery time in minutes (Mean ± SD)	52 ± 8	57 ± 9	0.001
Duration of surgery in minutes (Mean ± SD)	227 ± 12	233 ± 13	0.005

Table 2.
Postoperative characteristics.

Variable	Diabetic (n = 116)	Non-diabetic (n = 94)	Difference	95% CI
Post-operative IABP	2 (1.7%)	1(1.1%)	0.6	-4.3 - 5.0
Atrial fibrillation	12 (10.4%)	8(8.8%)	1.6	-7.0 - 9.7
Post-operative stroke	0	0		
Diaphragmatic paralysis	0	1(1.1%)	1.1	-2.2 - 5.8
Pleural effusion	1(0.9%)	2(2.1%)	1.2	-2.9 - 6.5
Hospital acquired pneumonia	2(1.7%)	1(1.1%)	0.6	-4.3 - 5.0
Low cardiac output	2(1.7%)	1(1.1%)	0.6	-4.3 - 5.0
Bleeding re-operation	0	0		
ICU stay in day (mean)	4	3	1.0	0.6 - 1.4

Table 3.
Postoperative morbidity.

Variable	Diabetic (n = 116)	Non-diabetic (n = 94)	Difference	95% CI
Superficial Wound Infection	2(1.7%)	1(1.1%)	0.6	-4.3 - 5.0
Deep sternal wound infection	0	0	NA	
Mortality	2(1.7%)	1(1.1%)	0.6	-4.3 - 5.0

Table 4.
Postoperative infection and the mortality rate.

in non-diabetic patients. Two-hundred and ten patients who underwent CABG using bilateral internal thoracic arteries were enrolled in the study and were divided into two groups: group I diabetic patients (DM) (n = 116) and group II non-diabetic patients (non-DM) patients (n = 94) (**Tables 1–4**).

3. Surgical procedures

All patients were disinfected with dermic isobetadine (iso-Betadine Dermique, 10% solution, povidone iodine) on their whole body. A lateral drape with plastic protector was used. All procedures were performed via median sternotomy. IMAs were harvested in a skeletonized fashion since only the artery is carefully dissected off the chest wall. Once upon completion of harvesting, IMAs were prepared with papaverine.

Extracorporeal circulation (ECC) was used in 78 patients whereas off-pump CABG was performed in 132 patients.

Combinations and numbers of arterial bypasses were selected according to the angiographic findings. When the bilateral internal mammary artery (BIMA) was grafted in situ, the left internal mammary artery (LIMA) was generally used for the left descending artery (LAD) and the RIMA for the lateral wall, usually going In Situ. In 38 patients having a Y-graft, the left coronary system was chosen as the target site of revascularization and a saphenous graft was used if necessary. The mean number of distal anastomosis was 2.6.

Before sternal closure, mediastinum was irrigated with warm saline and topical Vancomycin was routinely applied. Interlocking Multi-twisted closure sternal technique was used (**Table 2**).

4. Data analysis

Statistical Package for Social and Sciences (SPSS) version was used for data management. Descriptive data analysis was performed and data were presented in number (n) and percentages (%). Mean ± SD was reported for continuous variables. Statistical signıficance difference was assessed by using T-test for continuous variables and Chi squared for categorical variables and proportion, *P* value of (<0.05) was considered significant [2, 3].

5. Results

We included 210 patients, men (n = 200) and women (n = 10). The median age was 52.1 +/−9 years, 116 patients were DM and 100 patients of them in insulin, the median BMI was 29.1+/−4.6 kg/m^2 and the mean Euro SCORE was 4.8.

Overall operative mortality was 2.8% and was recorded in three high risk patients with severe LV systolic dysfunction (ejection fraction < 30%).

No statistical difference between the two groups was observed. There were no stroke or transient neurologic accident happened among our patients even no reoperation for bleeding (**Table 3**).

Deep sternal wound infection occurred in none off our patients. Only three cases showed signs of superficial wound infection that healed promptly following daily dressing, antibiotics and strict glycemic control (**Table 4**).

6. Discussion

Since 1980s, internal mammary artery (IMA) has become the graft of choice, thanks to clinical and angiographic data showing its long term patency rates and its superiority over the saphenous vein graft. Subsequently, the use of more arterial grafts especially bilateral mammary arteries was studied to achieve better long-term results when compared to single IMA and SVG. Interestingly, many analyses have demonstrated that patients undergoing CABG with bilateral internal mammary artery (BIMA) grafting have significantly improved survival and freedom from repeat revascularization when compared with patients receiving a single internal mammary artery (SIMA) [4].

Accordingly, the use of BIMA in diabetics was studied as long as CABG has emerged as the best option of myocardial revascularization in this group [5]. However, in spite of Histological superiority of IMA and the improved outcomes, the use of BIMA in patients with diabetes mellitus is still debated mainly due to the higher risk of sternal infection which remains a life-threatening complication after cardiac surgery associated with increased morbidity and mortality.

The ART trial is the first randomized study that compares outcome of single and bilateral internal thoracic artery grafting for CABG. Survival after BIMA versus SIMA grafting is being assessed by the randomized controlled Arterial Revascularization Trial (ART) [6]. Analysis of early data from this trial demonstrated similar surgical mortality and major morbidity for both the SIMA and the BIMA groups at 30 days and 1 year but with a small increase in the need for sternal wound reconstruction using BIMA. In our study BIMA used in selected diabetic patients do not lead to a significant higher incidence of deep sternal wound infection. We did not get the late survival advantage of using both internal thoracic arteries in this cohort. These results support the feasibility of CABG using BIMA grafts in patients undergoing CABG however Special cautions should to use BIMA in diabetics have been highlighted [7, 8].

Recently, it has been suggested that the skeletonization technique of internal thoracic artery reduces the risk of deep sternal wound complications by preserving sternal vascularization. Furthermore, a recent meta-analysis compared the incidence of sternal wound infection in diabetic patients undergoing skeletonized and pedicled IMA harvest. While pedicled BIMA harvest clearly increases the risk of DSWI, skeletonized BIMA harvest can be safely performed in diabetic patients [6].

Similarly, other measures should be applied in order to reduce the risk of sternal wound infection especially in diabetic patients. A recent prospective study showed the importance of a tight glycemic control with continuous intravenous insulin infusion- in comparison with fractional subcutaneous insulin injections, reduces significantly serum glucose levels and leads to a significant reduction in deep sternal wound infection rates [9]. Other studies highlighted that patients receiving topical vancomycin before closure of the incision had less superficial sternal infections (0% vs. 1.6%; $P < 0.0001$), deep sternal infections (0% vs. 0.7%; $P = 0.005$), any type of sternal infection (0% vs. 2.2%; $P < .0001$) and more interestingly a significant decrease in sternal infections of any type in patients with diabetes mellitus (0% vs. 3.3%; $P = 0.0004$). As a conclusion they mentioned that topical vancomycin applied to the sternal edges, in conjunction with perioperative antibiotics and controlled glycemic level, helps to eliminate wound infections in cardiac surgical patients [10].

Contraindications to bilateral IMAs, according to the ART Trial, would be insulin-dependent diabetes mellitus, specifically in obese individuals, and chronic obstructive airways disease with some early shoots of higher complications in women and the elderly, which were thus relative contraindications [11]. Nevertheless, our protocol reveals that the feasibility of the double mammary in insulin -dependent diabetic patients without affecting the incidence of deep sternal wound infection, in condition with tight glycemic control and strict hygiene during perioperative period.

7. Conclusions

Excellent outcomes following BIMA grafting can be expected in diabetic patients with a similar morbimortality compared to non-diabetic patients. Thus, use of BIMA grafting is an acceptable surgical procedure technique for diabetic patients. It provides multiple grafting with the best arterial conduits (IMAs) and is associated with an acceptable risk of deep sternal infections provided that preventive measures are taken. Indeed, adherence to a policy of strict perioperative glycemic control, good surgical technique, skeletonization, as well as effective post-operative management of surgical wounds would maximize the adoption of BIMA grafting as a default revascularization strategy even for diabetic patients. Further randomized controlled trials with longer follow-up are needed to confirm the safety and efficiency of BIMA grafting in diabetics.

Author details

Hassane Abdallah[1]*, Ahmed Ibrahim[2] and Khalid Al Khamees[3]

1 Consultant Cardiac Surgeon, Cardiac Surgery Department, Prince Sultan Cardiac Center, AlHassa, Saudi Arabia

2 Consultant Epidemiologist, Research and Biostatistics Department, Prince Sultan Cardiac Center, AlHassa, Saudi Arabia

3 Consultant Cardiac Surgeon, Chairman Cardiac Surgery, Director of VAD Program, CEO- Prince Sultan Cardiac Center, AlHassa, Saudi Arabia

*Address all correspondence to: abdallahhassane@hotmail.com

References

[1] Global Health Estimates 2016: Deaths by Cause, Age, Sex, by Country and by Region. 2000- 2016. Geneva, Switzerland: World Health Organization; 2018. Available from http://www.who.int/healthinfo/global_burden_disease/estimates/en/. [Accessed from: 28 October 2019]

[2] Ltman DG. Statistics with Confidence. In: Hopkins W, Batterham AM, editors. Bristol: BMJ Books; 2000;**49**:6

[3] Campbell I. Chi-squared and Fisher-Irwin tests of two-by-two tables with small sample recommendations. Statistics in Medicine. 2007;**26**:3661-3675

[4] Yi G, Shine B, Rehman SM, Altman DG, Taggart DP. Effect of bilateral internal mammary artery grafts on long-term Survival: A meta-analysis approach. Circulation. 2014;**130**:539-545

[5] Edwin L. Alderman, Katharine Andrews, James Bost, Martial Bourassa et al. Comparison of coronary artery bypass surgery with angioplasty in patients with multivessel disease. The bypass angioplasty revascularization Investi- gation (BARI) investigators. The New England Journal of Medicine. 1996;**335**:217-225

[6] Taggart D, Altman D, Gray A, Lees B, Nugara F, Yu L, et al. ART investigators. Randomized trial to compare bilateral vs. single internal mammary in coronary artery bypass grafting: 1-year results of the arterial revascularisation trial (ART). European Heart Journal. 2010;**31**:2470-2481

[7] Taggart DP et al. Randomized trial of bilateral versus single internal-thoracic-artery grafts. The New England Journal of Medicine. 2016;**375**(26):2540-2549. DOI: 10.1056/NEJMoa1610021

[8] Kelly R, Buth K, Legare JF. Bilateral internal thoracic artery grafting is superior to other forms of multiple arterial grafting in providing survival after coronary bypass surgery. The Journal of Thoracic and Cardiovascular Surgery. 2012;**144**:1408e15

[9] Furnary AP, Zerr KJ, Grunkemeier GL, Starr A. Continuous intravenous insulin infusion reduces the incidence of deep sternal wound infection in diabetic patients after cardiac surgical procedures. The Annals of Thoracic Surgery. 1999;**67**(2):352-362

[10] Lazar HL, Ketchedjian A, Haime M, Karlson K, Cabral H. Topical vancomycin in combination with perioperative antibiotics and tight glycemic control helps to eliminate sternal wound infections. The Journal of Thoracic and Cardiovascular Surgery. 2014 Sep;**148**(3):1035-1038. 1038-1040. DOI: 10.1016/j.jtcvs.2014.06.045

[11] Taggart DP, Benedetto U, Gerry S, Altman DG, Gray AM, Lees B, et al Bilateral versus single internal thoracic artery grafts at 10 years. The New England Journal of Medicine 2019;380:437-446

Chapter 8

Right Internal Thoracic Artery with an Anteroaortic Course

Maurilio O. Deininger, Orlando G. Oliveira, Daniel M.S. Magalhães and Eugenia Di G. Deininger

Abstract

Coronary artery bypass graft surgery remains the procedure of choice to revascularize patients with complex multivessel coronary artery disease. The left internal thoracic artery and saphenous vein are the most commonly utilized conduits in coronary artery bypass graft surgery. The left internal thoracic artery is widely accepted as the conduit of choice for coronary artery bypass grafting. Accumulated evidence in recent years has demonstrated the superiority of bilateral internal thoracic artery grafting over single internal thoracic artery grafting in terms of event-free survival, freedom from reintervention and survival. The survival benefit seen with bilateral internal thoracic artery grafting has been associated particularly with grafting the myocardium supplied by the left coronary artery system. Many surgical strategies have been tested in order to achieve left-sided myocardial revascularization with bilateral internal thoracic artery grafting. These include directing the right internal thoracic artery through the transverse sinus in a retroaortic course, free graft connected proximally either to the left internal thoracic artery (composite grafting) or to the ascending aorta. Another technical option is in situ right internal thoracic artery to the left anterior descending and left internal thoracic artery to circumflex marginal branches; in this chapter we will comment on this technique.

Keywords: bilateral internal thoracic artery, coronary artery bypass grafting, right internal thoracic artery, myocardial revascularization, coronary artery disease

1. Introduction

The treatment of coronary artery disease (CAD) is one of the most studied topics in medicine. Surgery for coronary artery bypass grafting (CABG) remains an excellent therapeutic option for the management of obstructive CAD, even with the development of new drugs and better results obtained with percutaneous treatment [1].

Although the saphenous vein is still widely used for aortic/coronary graft, due to the ease of harvest, preparation, and its use for making multiple grafts, this graft may develop intimal hyperplasia and atherosclerotic lesion, with occlusion rates of 10–15% in the first year after surgery; still, after one decade only 60% of vein grafts are patent, and of these only 50% are free of significant stenosis. Among some causes for the failure of the graft, we can cite the presence of valves in the veins and the risk of dilatation (varicosities). In addition to this, complications may occur in the lower limb where its harvest was performed. The internal thoracic artery (ITA) rarely develops atherosclerosis, and its diameter is normally compatible with coronary artery to be revascularized [2].

Recently, several studies corroborate the superiority of the use of both internal thoracic arteries (ITAs) instead of the use of only one, especially the use of the left internal thoracic artery (LITA) to the left anterior descending branch (LAD), considered to be the gold standard in CABG as a consequence of the excellent long-term patency. However, the use of right internal thoracic artery (RITA) offers similar results to those obtained with the use of LITA when used for the LAD [1, 3]. Some authors consider that RITA is better as a second arterial graft than the radial artery (RA), particularly in relation to the occurrence of cardiac events such as perioperative myocardial infarction (MI) as a consequence of vasospasm, which can occur in up to 10% of patients [4].

The use of RITA for the right coronary artery (RCA) and its branches showed different results when compared to using left coronary (LC) system, with patency similar to the saphenous vein. For this reason, RITA became more used for LC as a compound graft with the LITA, also as a free graft, or at retroaortic position for branches of the circumflex coronary artery (CX) [3], and another alternative strategy is in situ RITA to LAD [1, 3, 5, 6].

Complete revascularization with arterial grafting shows better long-term outcomes after CABG. The superiority of the ITAs compared to other arterial grafts is already well accepted with excellent long-term results as can be seen widely in the literature [7].

2. Right internal thoracic artery with an anteroaortic course

Rene Favaloro published his first paper in April 1968 describing CABG surgery [8]. Since then, CABG has been with no doubt the most widely studied surgical procedure. But one important controversy that persists until now is about the ideal graft for revascularization, and mainly, whether the use of multiple arterial grafts results in significant improvement in long-term outcomes.

Multiple arterial conduits are used aiming to reduce the likelihood of future reoperations, especially both ITAs. But, there is still a fear of using both ITAs in some subgroups of patients, such as elderly, obese, and diabetic. However, some authors have observed that the skeletonization of ITAs and CABG surgery when performed without cardiopulmonary bypass (CPB) cause a reduction in the incidence of sternal infection. This benefit is more evident in diabetic patients, where there may be a 60% reduction in the occurrence of this complication, allowing removal of both ITAs, without offering additional risk for infectious complications of the sternum [9, 10]. Others noted that the use of pedicled ITA and CPB are independent risk factors for mediastinitis in surgery for CABG [11].

When we use the antegrade RITA, in single or sequential graft, for the LAD territory, we could use the LITA to the territory of CX. With this technique the entire left coronary system is revascularized with arterial grafts only (RITA and LITA), all in situ. To turn this surgery into a frequent treatment possible, the RITA to the anterior region of the heart needs to show the same good results as the LITA when used for its purpose, a result confirmed by a randomized study conducted by us [1]. **Figure 1** shows details using the two ITAs for the territory of the left coronary artery and video 1 available from https://www.dropbox.com/s/0p2mcch5qw67clf/Video%201%20-%20Animation%20RITA%20and%20LITA.mp4?dl=0 (animation showing the use of both ITAs for the left coronary artery).

On the other hand, if we use the ITA combined with another compound graft, with "Y" anastomosis, for example, all the blood flowing to the grafted coronary

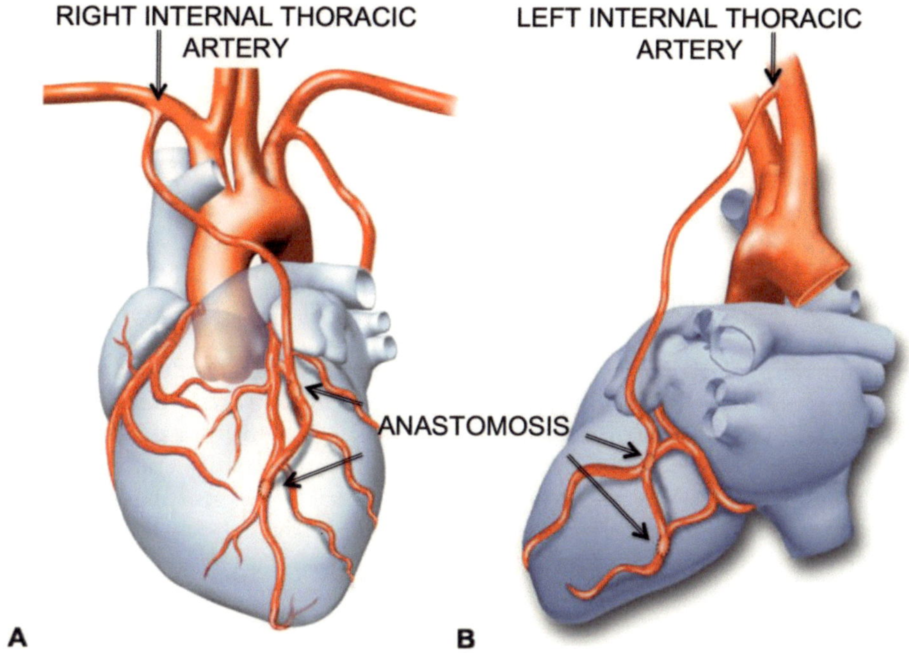

Figure 1.
(A) This schematic drawing shows the anterior view of the heart with the RITA being used anterograde, in sequential anastomosis for diagonal and LAD coronaries. (B) Lateral view of the heart showing LITA being used in situ, in sequential anastomosis for two left marginal branches. RITA: Right internal thoracic artery; LAD: left anterior descending; LITA: left internal thoracic artery.

ends up being from only one source of supply, usually the LITA. A reduction in its flow, due to spasm, can result in drastic consequences such as global ischemia of the left coronary territory [12].

We performed a randomized prospective study where we evaluated the patency of the LITA compared to the RITA when used for the territory of the anterior interventricular branch. The aim of this technique is to use the antegrade RITA, in single or sequential graft, for the LAD territory, and to use the LITA to the territory of CX. Due to the good long-term results when using both ITAs and to the fact that, as a consequence, the entire left coronary system is revascularized with arterial grafts only, i.e., RITA and LITA, all in situ, allowing two sources of blood supply, this could reduce the chance of reoperation for a new myocardial revascularization.

The primary aim of our study was to assess the patency of the pedicled RITA used in CABG, in the anteroaortic position in anastomosis to the LAD compared with LITA used in the same position. The secondary aim was to assess the occurrence of death or cardiac events such as myocardial infarction (MI) and recurrent angina or need for reintervention (reoperation for CABG or coronary angioplasty), as well as to assess the patency of other grafts. The patency was evaluated by multislice coronary angiotomography at the sixth postoperative month.

This study project was presented and approved by the Ethics and Research Committee of the Lauro Wanderley University Hospital, which belongs to Federal University of Paraíba, and Ethics Committee for Analysis of Research Projects (CAPPesq) of the Clinical Board of the Clinics Hospital and the Faculty of Medicine of the University of São Paulo, with the research protocol number 0844/08, CAPPesq, December 17, 2008. This project was performed with the approval of these committees and under the supervision of the Surgical Unit of Coronary Surgery Division of Heart Institute at Clinics Hospital of the Faculty of Medicine, University of São Paulo.

For randomization purposes, patients or guardians have to agree and sign the written informed consent, after being informed of it by a staff member. This study involved 100 patients who underwent cardiac surgery for off-pump coronary artery bypass (OPCAB), prospectively, randomized by computer before the beginning of the study. The surgeon knew the selected group only at the beginning of surgery, that is, which graft would be placed in the LAD territory (RITA or LITA). Patients did not know which technique would be used. The number of patients was calculated according to the probability of a difference of 15% occlusion higher than the standard, LITA to the LAD, for a value of probability error of 0.05 and a power of 80% sample with P of 0.05%.

There was no conflict of interest of any of the researchers involved in this research project.

Patients were selected after doing coronary angiographies. These exams were evaluated by at least two surgeons and should reveal coronary artery disease in at least two vessels of the left coronary artery territory with significant stenosis (> 70%), presenting angina (stable or unstable) and left ventricular ejection fraction (LV-EF) higher than 30%. Patients with coronary artery bypass grafting combined with another procedure, circulatory assistance for cardiogenic shock, the use of intra-aortic balloon pump, LV-EF less than 30%, and reoperations were excluded. Obese or diabetic patients were not excluded; age limit has not been established. Since these criteria have been fulfilled, the patient was selected and invited to participate in the research. In order to provide similarity between the groups, we draw two strategies for the use of BITA and allocated patients in Group-1 (G-1) and Group-2 (G-2), both with 50 randomized patients. The patency of the right and left internal thoracic arteries was comparatively studied.

In G-1, LITA was used in situ with anastomosis to LAD (single or sequential anastomosis), and complementing revascularization with the free RITA to the CX territory, used in sequential anastomosis when needed, and another graft to the RC territory (saphenous vein or RA). In G-2, RITA was used in situ, anterograde with anastomosis to LAD (single or sequential anastomosis) and complementing revascularization with LITA; also in situ for the CX territory, used in sequential anastomosis when needed; and another graft to the RC territory (saphenous vein or RA). Video 2 is available from https://www.dropbox.com/s/e1g89hucaukjv0z/Video%202%20-%20RITA%20Sequencial%20anastomosis.mp4?dl=0 (demonstrating technical details of the sequential anastomosis from RITA to LAD and diagonal artery).

Clinical aspects were cataloged during the preoperative period to assess the similarity between the two groups. The occurrence of perioperative MI was assessed considering ST segment elevation greater than 1 mm at the limb leads or 2 mm at precordial leads at least two contiguous leads or some area of necrosis that did not exist at preoperative ECG. We also analyzed elevation of creatine kinase-MB (CK-MB) above 100 IU/l and troponin I level above 2.5 ng/mL within 48 hours after surgery.

To assess the coronary graft patency, patients of both groups were submitted to multislice CT angiography studies with 128 channels at 6 months after surgery. We used a Philips CT scanner (Brilliance CT), with schemes of 120 kV and 800–1000 mA of irradiation; 0.67 mm cuts were performed, using wherever possible the 75% stage. The time of apnea to capture images was around 15 seconds. In patients with heart rate (HR) above 65 beats per minute (bpm), a beta-blocker (metoprolol) at a dose of 2.5–15 mg (titrating to achieve HR less than 65 bpm) was used. Since patients had already undergone coronary artery bypass grafting, calcium score was not performed.

We performed median sternotomy. Special attention was given to the pericardiotomy; it was opened longitudinally, between the ascending aorta and the superior vena cava, where we made a tunnel through the thymic fat for the passage of the ATID. The ATIs were dissected using skeletonization and used in situ for the LAD territory depending on the group that was allocated. **Figures 2** and **3** show details of the opening of the pericardium and RITA's positioning. Video 3 available from https://www.dropbox.com/s/4myr68cb1lfu3m8/Video%203%20-%20Opening%20of%20the%20pericardium.mp4?dl=0 shows surgical technical detail.

Initially we performed the anastomosis of the ATI to LAD (single or sequential anastomosis), then we performed the anastomosis (saphenous or radial artery) to RC artery territory. This strategy provides more security to bring the heart medially and expose the sidewall. Sometimes this maneuver can lead to hemodynamic instability. For better exposure of the coronary arteries, we used Lima's point [13], suction stabilizer, and intracoronary shunt to allow more comfort during anastomosis.

The RITA was positioned across the mediastinum anteriorly. We made a tunnel using blunt dissection through the pericardial and pleural fat, anterior to the right phrenic nerve at the most cranial portion of the aorta. This way, the RITA is covered with mediastinal fat, previously isolated, making a tunnel on the aorta, allowing the RITA to stay on the free space between the aorta and the sternum, eliminating

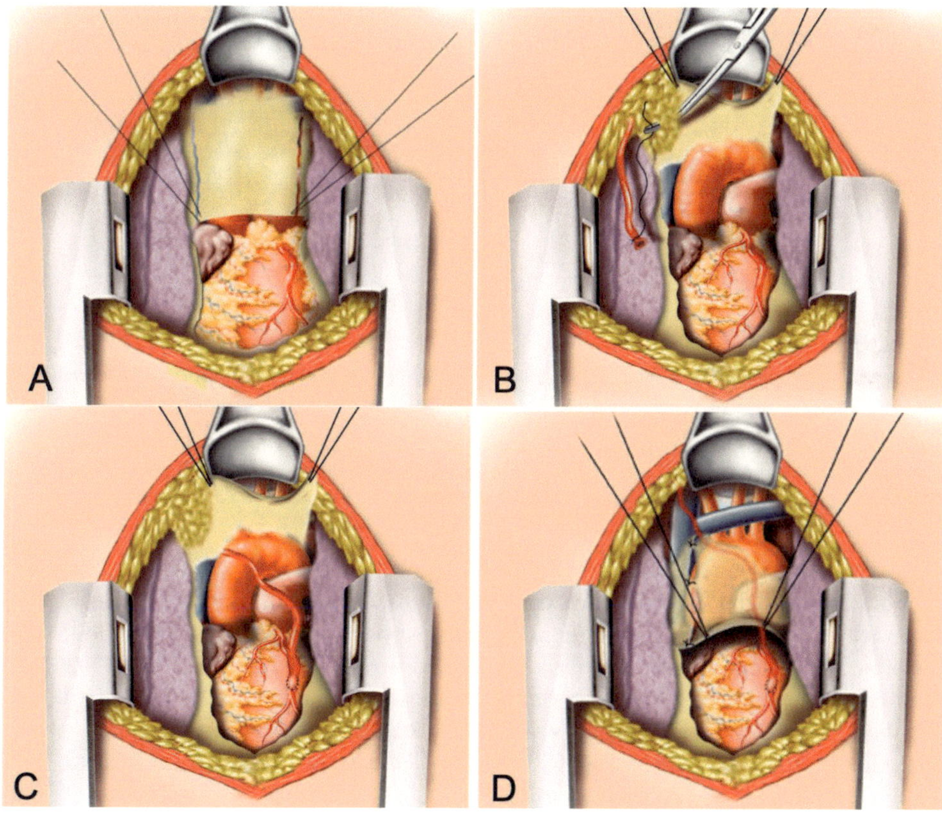

Figure 2.
(A) Schematic drawing showing the preservation of the pericardium and adjacent fat tissue, which will be used later to cover the RITA when crossing the mediastinum at the level of the ascending aorta. (B) Schematic drawing showing the pericardium and the adjacent tissue being used to perform a tunnel with a clamp through the mediastinal fat to pass the RITA. (C) Schematic drawing showing the pericardium and adjacent fat tissue, being moved aside to show the RITA after anastomosis to the LAD. (D) Drawing showing the RITA crossing the mediastinum and being covered by the mediastinal fat, preventing it from adhering to the sternum bone. RITA: Right internal thoracic artery; LAD: left anterior descending.

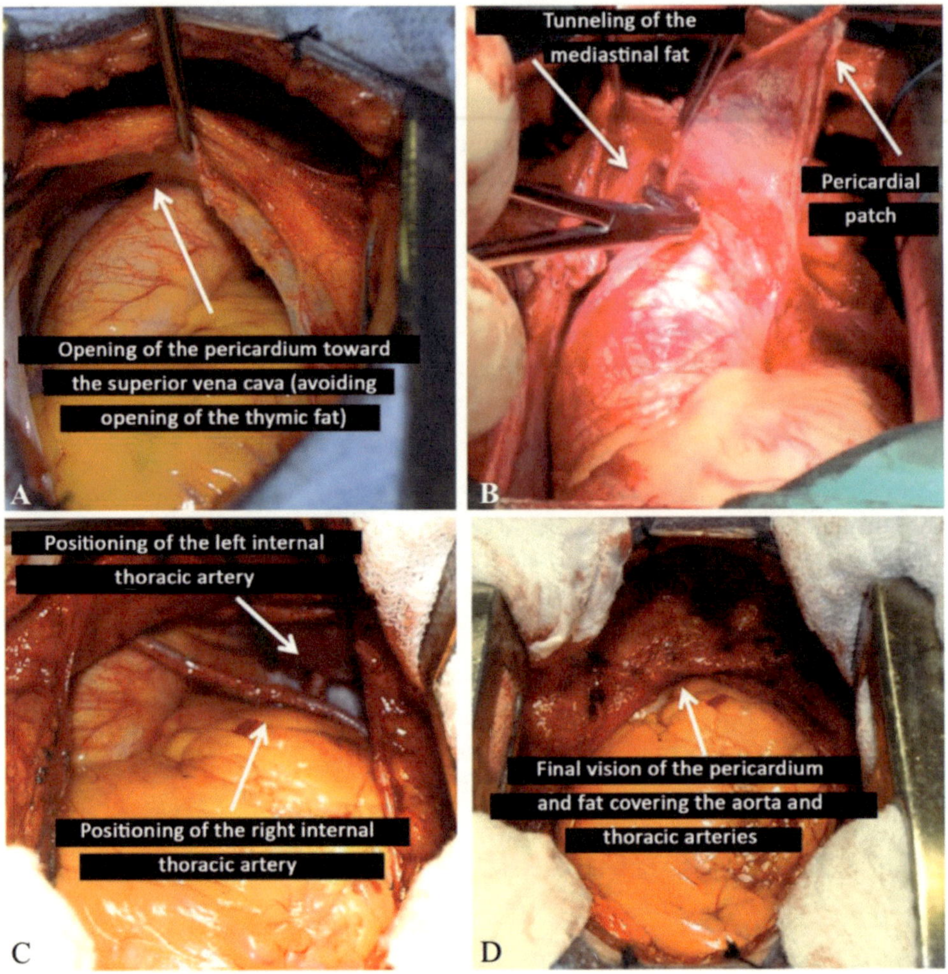

Figure 3.
(A) Surgical photo showing the opening of the pericardium until the limit of the superior vena cava, preserving all the thymic fat. (B) Surgical photo showing the pericardium being moved aside to performing a tunnel with clamp. (C) Surgical photo showing the positioning of the RITA crossing the mediastinum through the mediastinal fat and positioned on the cranial portion of the ascending aorta. A small segment of LITA is seen penetrating the pericardial cavity through a window on the left lateral side of the pericardium. (D) Surgical photo showing the final view where mediastinal fat and pericardium cover the entire ascending aorta and RITA. RITA: Right internal thoracic artery; LITA: left internal thoracic artery.

the possibility of the first to attach the latter. **Figures 4** and **5** show multislice coronary angiotomography images showing the positioning of the RITA. Video 4 available from https://www.dropbox.com/s/0vwao9267x3fd71/Video%204%20%20Tunnel%20through%20the%20pericardial%20and%20pleural%20fat.mp4?dl=0 and video 5 available from https://www.dropbox.com/s/lfa2b8xdf4kv7mc/Video%205%20-%20Positioning%20of%20RITA%20and%20LITA.mp4?dl=0, demonstrating surgical technical details.

High levels of troponin I after CABG do not necessarily indicate that the graft is occluded, but only that there was a significant myocardial injury during or after the procedure. We performed off-pump surgery in 95% of patients in this series. In several patients we performed four arterial anastomoses to LC artery territory, which was possibly due to the sequential anastomosis using both ITAs. This shows that with a good surgical strategy, it is possible to perform a full OPCAB using both ITAs [1].

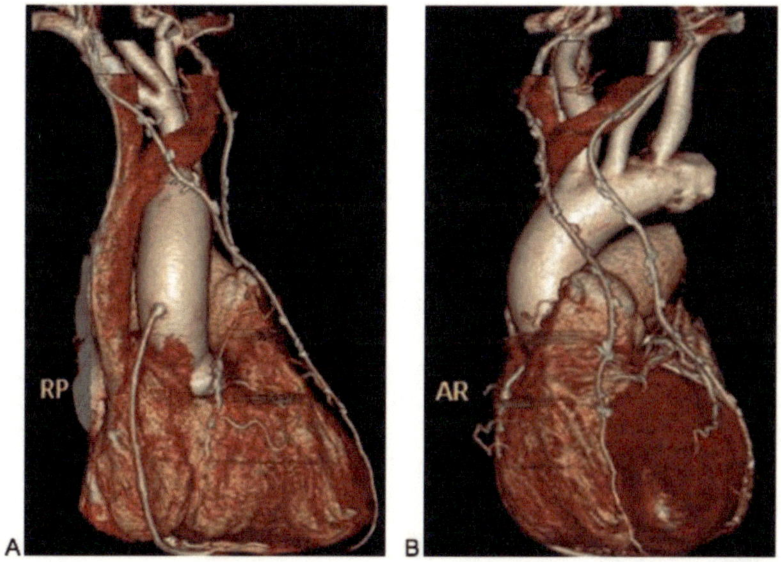

Figure 4.
(A) Multislice coronary angiotomography image shows the RITA position at cranial portion of the ascending aorta, anastomosed to the LAD, and saphenous vein graft anastomosis to the posterior descending artery. (B) Multislice coronary angiotomography image shows the RITA position at the cranial portion of the ascending aorta, anastomosis to the left anterior descending, and LITA anastomosis to the left marginal branch. RITA: Right internal thoracic artery; LAD: left anterior descending; LITA: left internal thoracic artery.

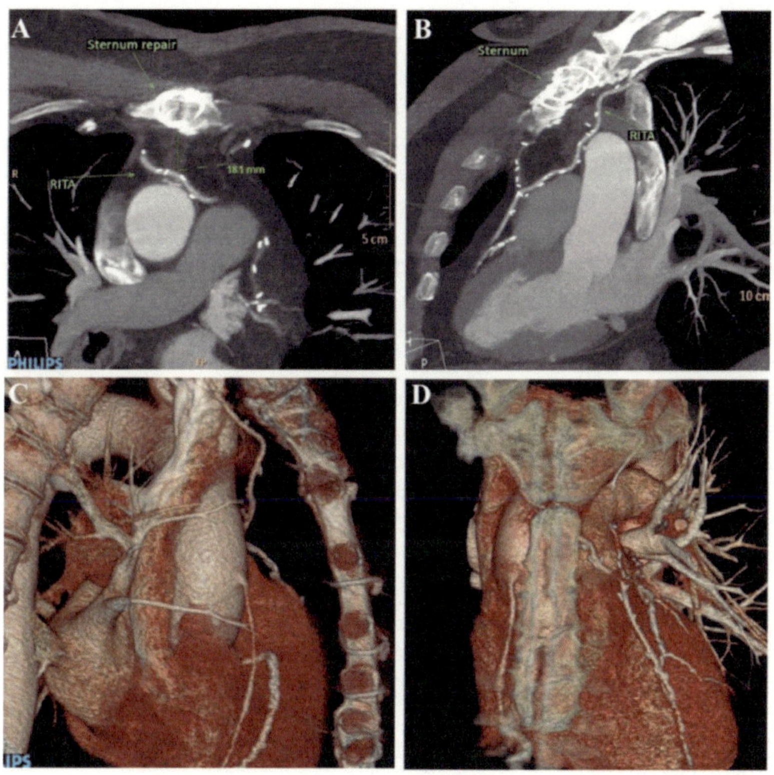

Figure 5.
(A) and (B) Multislice coronary angiotomography images show the positioning of the RITA highlighting its distance from the sternum (18.1 mm). (C) and (D) Multislice coronary angiotomography images show the positioning of the RITA at the cranial portion of the ascending aorta anastomosed to the left anterior descending. We also observe the saphenous vein graft to the posterior descending artery.

The primary endpoint was the graft patency of ITAs used to graft the LAD, and the secondary endpoint was the occurrence of death or cardiac events such as MI, recurrent angina, and need for reoperation. The observation period was 6 months after surgery until angiotomography was performed. For statistical analysis, Chi-square and Fisher's exact test were used to compare proportions and Student's t-test for numeric values with results expressed as mean and standard deviation. The software used was GraphPad Prism 5.2.

There was no death in any group, nor any permanent neurological complication, or need for revascularization, percutaneous or surgical, in any patient in the two groups during the observation period of 6 months. Multislice coronary angiotomography was performed at 6 months after surgery in 96 of the 100 patients. None of the ITAs (RITA or LITA), grafted in LAD, showed occlusion or stenosis [1].

After the good results obtained with this technique, we started to use it routinely. We already use RITA for the territory of the LAD branch and LIMA for the circumflex territory in more than 1500 patients.

3. Comment

Despite the good results, this surgery is not frequently used in major centers around the world. It is known that, in addition to the fear of the risk of sternal infection or severe bleeding, using both ITAs increases surgical time and requires more refined technique. As there are still doubts and controversies regarding the best surgical strategy, the use of both ITAs is still not routinely performed in all services and in all subgroups of patients. Consequently, the utilization rates of ITAs range from 4 to 30%, even in countries like the USA, Japan, and some European countries [14]. Evidence clearly shows the superiority of the use of both ITAs in CABG surgery. Evidence from observational studies is being incorporated into the guidelines of cardiac surgery societies, making the use of arterial grafts recommended in CABG by the American and European guidelines and in a more recent position paper by the Society of Thoracic Surgeons [15].

Some authors showed that the use of anteroaortic RITA or LITA has similar patency when grafted to the LAD [1, 16, 17]. When we use anteroaortic RITA to LAD, this technique allows the entire left coronary system to be revascularized with two independent sources of blood supply, using both ITAs in situ, that is, RITA for LAD territory and LITA for CX territory. However, one of the limitations for the use of this technique is the crossing of the mediastinum by the ATID, which may cause graft injury in the case of reoperation, due to the risk of the ATID adhering to the sternum. To minimize this risk, some authors advocate the use of a PTFE tube or a pedicled thymic fat to protect the LITA when crossing the mediastinum [1, 5]. Another limitation to the use of RITA to LAD is the difficulty to achieve the desired anastomosis site, in the event of the need to perform a distal anastomosis. Based on some authors' experience, this limitation occurs in 6% of the cases, and, in these cases, a RITA "Y" composite graft with LITA can be performed [1]. When we use the skeletonized ITA, the length of this artery increases compared to the pedicle artery, thus allowing RITA to reach the LAD (20.1 vs. 16.4 cm, $P < 0.001$.); in addition there was a reduction of infectious complications in the diabetic patients' sternum (2.2 vs. 10.0%, $P < 0.05$) [18]. The reduction of the risk of sternal osteomyelitis with this technique is due to the preservation of the blood supply and lymphatic drainage, and consequently leading to increased flow compared to the non-skeletonized ITA [7].

Some authors observed that using saphenous vein graft for the RC territory brings results as satisfactory as RITA for that same region of the heart [5, 6].

The long-term benefit can be obtained when both ITAs are used to irrigate the LC territory [1, 19, 20]. The other option to use both in situ ITAs to the left coronary system is the retroaortic RITA for CX territory [4, 7]. However, some authors cite limitations on using this technique because the RITA length cannot reach two or three LM branches for sequential anastomosis, especially in off-pump surgery. When we use this technique and the CABG is performed without CPB, the confection of this anastomosis is impaired by the need to bring the heart to expose the coronary branches of lateral wall, distancing the coronary artery from the graft. On the other hand, at anteroaortic position this mentioned difficulty does not occur. The course of retroaortic RITA may present some disadvantages, such as difficulty to control the bleed of any branch or aortic artery compression or kinks not detected [20]. Another technique that can be used is bilateral ITA in "Y" composite graft (free RITA joined to the side of the LITA). Video 6 available from https://www.dropbox.com/s/c71rbgpy7bzfwjs/Video%206%20%20%22Y%22anastomosis.mp4?dl=0 shows coronaryography of a patient undergoing this technique. A meta-analysis of the studies comparing in situ with "Y" graft ITA configurations showed no significant difference in clinical outcomes [21].

The presentation and publication in November 2016 of the planned 5-year interim analysis (of 10-year survival, a primary outcome) of the Arterial Revascularization Trial (ART) of the American Heart Association left the community of cardiac surgeons around the world surprised. The trial ART is the largest randomized study using arterial grafts, involving 28 centers in 7 countries and 3102 patients randomized to receive single internal thoracic arteries (SITAs) or bilateral internal thoracic arteries (BITAs). There are several potential limitations to ART trial, for example, near 20% of patients receiving a SITA graft also received a radial artery graft, which may have further narrowed any potential differences between SITA and BITA [22]. Despite these limitations, ART trial remains the most solid available evidence comparing SITA versus BITA grafts. Furthermore, although the results of ART trial contradict much of the results of published observational studies, they are consistent with Cleveland Clinic results of nearly 20 years ago reporting a survival benefit of BITA grafts after 5 years; this benefit becomes more evident over the years [23].

After evaluating ITA remodeling, some authors cite predictors of occlusion: large accessory branches leading to theft of flow, flow through the native coronary bed, and quality of the distal coronary bed. When using both ITAs, the best results are obtained when they are used in the LC territory, preferably in occluded arteries or significant obstructive lesions. Patency is therefore determined by the flow competition, the nature of the graft, and the degree of stenosis of the coronary territory. Therefore, the graft deterioration is related to the degree of coronary branch obstruction when it is less than 75%. Competitive flow reduces the patency of arterial grafts after coronary bypass surgery. This competitive flow is dynamic, relative, and in a certain way inevitable. The preoperative assessment of the coronary stenosis severity and the prediction of competitive flow can be improved with the addition of fractional flow reserve (FFR) measurements to coronary angiography, but the potential for minimizing the effects of competitive flow by different graft configurations seems limited [24].

Regarding the CABG procedure itself, there is a significant gender differentiation, because only a small percentage of women receive complete arterial revascularization, as reported in the STS database (2.3% of women who underwent CABG from 2002 to 2005 received BITA grafting vs. 4.7% of men) [25]. Some authors do not use gender [1], obesity, or the presence of diabetes as exclusion criteria to use BITA grafting, but some consider females a risk factor, decreasing their chances to receive the best revascularization approach, BITA grafting. The long-term survival benefit of the systematic use of BITA grafting among women remains unclear. Lately, some authors have shown that women had a similar 10-year survival compared to men when BITA grafting was used. Others have shown that women who underwent CABG in which BITA grafting was used had better survival than the group that used SITA, especially in patients older than 65 years. Thus, it was demonstrated that the best results obtained with the use of BITA grafts are gender independent [26].

Several studies have shown that the use of bilateral in situ internal thoracic arteries provides excellent probabilities of event-free survival and cardiac event-free survival during follow-up of 15 and 20 years. More studies including elderly patients with severe comorbidities are needed. Results from studies with 15–20 years of total arterial revascularization suggest that cardiac surgeons should prefer total arterial grafts in order to reduce the risk of long-term cardiac events, especially during the second decade after surgery in relatively young and healthy patients. Despite the absence of a randomized control trial, there is evidence that the BITA graft is not only safe in the immediate postoperative period, but it has a supremacy over SITA use over long-term survival and absence of cardiac events. This is the reason why the use of RITA as a second arterial graft with LITA has acquired a Class IIa, evidence B indication at the European and American guidelines on myocardial revascularization [27, 28]. Total arterial revascularization using both ITAs is the best revascularization strategy that a cardiovascular community can offer for their patients with multivessel disease [29].

4. Conclusion

Coronary artery bypass grafting using antegrade in situ RITA for LAD territory, compared to the in situ LITA, anastomosed in the same region, presents the same results in an evaluation period of 6 months, assessed by multislice coronary angiotomography, as demonstrated by some authors [1]. The results demonstrated 100% grafts' patency. The OPCAB surgery that used both ITAs for LC territory proved to be safe, effective, and feasible, even in patients with multivessel disease.

The main reasons for the reluctance to use BITA grafts are its technical challenge, because it requires a high level of skill, experience, and concentration. The duration of surgeries is longer and may be associated with a minor increased risk of deep sternal wound infection in severe cases of diabetes, obesity, and/or chronic obstructive pulmonary disease. Another reason is the lack of convincing evidence of a randomized controlled trial. All these difficulties/problems can be overcome with the use of ITAs skeletonization. We should always bear in mind Lytle's statement made in 1999: "two internal thoracic artery grafts are better than one." Some studies already postulate the use of three arterial grafts in order to obtain better late survival.

The CABG off-pump surgery leads to less cell injury than the conventional method of CABG surgery (on-pump) [1, 10, 19]. Based on randomized and observational trials that have compared off- versus on-pump CABG, there is one point that most surgeons would agree with the following: surgeons have to be experienced and routinely use off-pump techniques to have comparable results with off- versus on-pump CABG. The best results with off-pump CABG come from centers with large volume of surgical patients [19].

Conflict of interest

The authors declare no conflict of interest.

Author details

Maurilio O. Deininger*, Orlando G. Oliveira, Daniel M.S. Magalhães and Eugenia Di G. Deininger
Alberto Urquisa Wanderley—Unimed Hospital, Sao Francisco Memorial Hospital, Joao Pessoa, Paraiba, Brazil

*Address all correspondence to: maurilio.od@gmail.com

References

[1] Deininger MO, Moreira LFP, Dallan LAO, Oliveira OG, Magalhães DMS, Deininer EG, et al. Comparative analysis of the patency of the internal thoracic artery in the CABG of left anterior descending artery: 6-month postoperative coronary CT angiography evaluation. Revista Brasileira de Cirurgia Cardiovascular. 2014;**29**(2):192-201

[2] Loop FD, Lytle BW, Cosgrove DM, Stewart RW, Goomastic M, Williams GW, et al. Influence of the internal-mammary-artery graft on 10-year survival and other cardiac events. The New England Journal of Medicine. 1986;**314**:1-6

[3] Raja SG. Surgical strategies for bilateral internal mammary artery grafting. International Journal of Surgery. 2015;**16**:140-145

[4] Ruttmann E, Fischler N, Sakic A, Chevtchik O, Alber H, Schistek R, et al. Second internal thoracic artery versus radial artery in coronary artery bypass grafting: A long-term, propensity score-matched follow-up study. Circulation. 2011;**124**(12):1321-1329

[5] Zacharias A. Protection of the right internal mammary artery in the retrosternal position with stented grafts. The Annals of Thoracic Surgery. 1995;**60**(6):1826-1828

[6] Lev-Ran O, Pevni D, Matsa M, Paz Y, Kramer A, Mohr R. Arterial myocardial revascularization with in situ crossover right internal thoracic artery to left anterior descending artery. The Annals of Thoracic Surgery. 2001;**72**(3):798-803

[7] Kurlansky PA, Traad EA, Dorman MJ, Galbut DL, Zucker M, Ebra G. Thirty- year follow-up defines survival benefit for second internal mammary artery in propensity-matched groups. The Annals of Thoracic Surgery. 2010;**90**:101-108

[8] Favaloro RG. Saphenous vein autograft replacement of severe segmental coronary artery occlusion. The Annals of Thoracic Surgery. 1968;**5**:334-339

[9] Saso S, James D, Vecht JA, Kidher E, Kokotsakis J, Malinovski V, et al. Effect of skeletonization of the internal thoracic artery for coronary revascularization on the incidence of sternal wound infection. The Annals of Thoracic Surgery. 2010;**89**(2):661-670

[10] Nakano J, Okabayashi H, Hanyu M, Soga Y, Nomoto T, Arai Y, et al. Risk factors for wound infection after off-pump coronary artery bypass grafting: Should bilateral internal thoracic arteries be harvested in patients with diabetes? The Journal of Thoracic and Cardiovascular Surgery. 2008;**135**(3):540-545

[11] Sá MPBO, Soares EF, Santos CA, Figueiredo OJ, Lima ROA, Escobar RR, et al. Fatores de risco para mediastinite após cirurgia de revascularização miocárdica. Revista Brasileira de Cirurgia Cardiovascular. 2011;**26**(1):27-35

[12] Paterson HS, Bannon PG. Composite Y grafts from the left internal mammary artery: Current considerations. Heart, Lung & Circulation. 2018;**27**(2):133-137

[13] Lima RC. Padronização técnica da revascularização do miocárdio da artéria circunflexa e seus ramos sem circulação extracorpórea [Tese de Doutorado]. São Paulo: Universidade Federal de São Paulo. Escola Paulista de Medicina; 1999

[14] Kinoshita T, Asai T. Bilateral internal thoracic artery grafting: Current state of the art. Innovations. 2011;**6**(2):77-83

[15] Aldea GS, Bakaeen FG, Pal J, Fremes S, Head SJ, Sabik J, et al. The Society of Thoracic Surgeons clinical practice guidelines on arterial conduits for coronary artery bypass grafting. The Annals of Thoracic Surgery. 2016;**101**:801-809

[16] Raja SG, Benedetto U, Husain M, Soliman R, De Robertis F, Amrani M, et al. Does grafting of the left anterior descending artery with the in situ right internal thoracic artery have an impact on late outcomes in the context of bilateral internal thoracic artery usage? The Journal of Thoracic and Cardiovascular Surgery. 2014;**148**:1275-1281

[17] Puskas JD, Yanagawa B, Taggart DP. Advancing the state of the art in surgical coronary revascularization. The Annals of Thoracic Surgery. 2016;**101**:419-421

[18] Calafiore AM, Vitolla G, Iaco AL, Fino C, Di Giammarco G, Marchesani F, et al. Bilateral internal mammary artery grafting: Midterm results of pedicled versus skeletonized conduits. The Annals of Thoracic Surgery. 1999;**67**(6):1637-1642

[19] Attia T, Halkos ME. Commentary: Reinventing the wheel: Off- versus on-pump redo coronary artery bypass grafting. The Journal of Thoracic and Cardiovascular Surgery. 2019. DOI: 10.1016/j.jtcvs.2019.04.100

[20] Shah PJ, Bui K, Blackmore S, Gordon I, Hare DL, Fuller J, et al. Has the in situ right internal thoracic artery been overlooked? An angiographic study of the radial artery, internal thoracic arteries and saphenous vein graft patencies in symptomatic patients. European Journal of Cardio-Thoracic Surgery. 2005;**27**(5):870-875

[21] Yanagawa B, Verma S, Jüni P, Tam DY, Mazine A, Puskas JD, et al. A systematic review and meta-analysis of in situ versus composite bilateral internal thoracic artery grafting. The Journal of Thoracic and Cardiovascular Surgery. 2017;**153**:1108-1116

[22] Taggart DP, Altman DG, Gray AM, Lees B, Gerry S, Benedetto U, et al. Randomized trial of bilateral versus single internal-thoracic- artery grafts. The New England Journal of Medicine. 2016;**375**:2540-2549

[23] Lytle BW, Blackstone EH, Loop FD, Houghtaling PL, Arnold JH, Akhrass R, et al. Two internal thoracic artery grafts are better than one. The Journal of Thoracic and Cardiovascular Surgery. 1999;**117**:855-872

[24] Paterson HS, Bannon PG, Taggart DP, et al. Competitive flow in coronary bypass surgery: The roles of fractional flow reserve and arterial graft configuration. The Journal of Thoracic and Cardiovascular Surgery. 2017;**154**:1570-1575

[25] Tabata M, Grab JD, Khalpey Z, Edwards FH, O'Brien SM, Cohn LH, et al. Prevalence and variability of internal mammary artery graft use in contemporary multivessel coronary artery bypass graft surgery: Analysis of the Society of Thoracic Surgeons national cardiac database. Circulation. 2009;**120**:935-940

[26] Vrancic JM, Navia DO, Espinoza JC, Piccinini F, Camporrotondo M, Benzadon M, et al. Is sex a risk factor for death in patients with bilateral internal thoracic artery grafts? The Journal of Thoracic and Cardiovascular Surgery. 2019. DOI: 10.1016/j.jtcvs.2019.01.025

[27] Windecker S, Kolh P, Alfonso F, Authors/Task Force Members, et al. 2014 ESC/EACTS guidelines on myocardial revascularization: The task force on myocardial revascularization of the European Society of Cardiology

(ESC) and the European Association for Cardio-Thoracic Surgery (EACTS) developed with the special contribution of the European Association of Percutaneous car- diovascular interventions (EAPCI). European Heart Journal. 2014;**35**(37):2541-2619

[28] Hillis LD, Smith PK, Anderson JL, et al. ACCF/AHA guideline for coronary artery bypass graft surgery: A report of the American College of Cardiology Foundation/American Heart Association task force on practice guidelines. Circulation. 2011;**124**(23):e652e735

[29] Davierwala PM, Mohr FW. Bilateral internal mammary artery grafting: Rationale and evidence. International Journal of Surgery. 2015;**16**:133-139

Chapter 9

Tips and Tricks in Microvascular Anastomoses

Sharifah Ahmad Roohi

Abstract

Microvascular anastomosis is a highly skilled surgical technique that requires the assistance of optical magnification via an operating microscope or loupes to be fully visualised and thus accomplished reasonably well. It demands the full attention of the surgeon throughout the procedure. Even the smallest of inadvertencies may result in disastrous results. Practice has no shortcut and the more experienced a **skilled** surgeon is, the better his results. The chapter begins with a detailed account of preparedness in the operating room, for preparation is the path to success. There are however tips to reduce the incline of the learning curve and points to remember when things are not quite going right. This chapter attempts to deal with those moments.

Keywords: arterial repair, microvascular anastomosis, replantation, revascularization techniques, venous repair and grafting

1. Introduction

Microvascular anastomosis is a fine art form which requires practice to get it perfect. Perfection is required to repair a vessel that is 2 mm or less in diameter with precision in order to prevent the development of a thrombus resulting in vessel occlusion. In order to achieve this, harmony should be present between the microscope, its operator (the surgeon), and his instruments. With experience, the surgeon may be able to successfully anastomose 1–2 mm diameter vessels with loupes magnification, but it is not recommended for the novice. This chapter is divided into two sections: the first is a **brief description** of the surgeon' s posture, his instruments, patient factors and the environment to illustrate how the harmony results in a better whole. In the second section, the **techniques** on how to accomplish the process without compromising the quality of repair and the **finer points** on how to enhance it will be highlighted to bring the whole orchestra to its crescendo and conclusion.

2. The components of the orchestra

There are four main components to the whole scenario. If we liken it to a Musical Concert, then the place where the whole operation takes place is the Operating Room (OR) while the main Conductor of the event is the Chief Surgeon. The surgical (musical) instruments are what are essential for the surgery to take place and finally the musical score is the patient upon which this whole event is dependent upon to be successful.

2.1 The operating room

The theatre where the drama takes place is the operating room. The environment in this room is critical to the success of the surgery. The conductor or Master of the OR is the surgeon and the environment should be tailored to his or her preference.

Microsurgery requires a steady hand and practiced skill. It takes hours to complete a replantation or undertake a coronary artery by-pass graft while demanding full concentration to the task at hand. Mundane issues must be sorted out for any discomfort may prolong the surgery and even render it unsuccessful.

2.1.1 Temperature and lighting

The temperature of the OR is of course controlled within specified limits of regulatory standards, but the main surgeon must be comfortable throughout the duration of the surgery.

The lighting, similarly, has to be of superb quality to visualise the most intricate detail. The aim is to have a well-illuminated field without shadows. The operating microscope achieves this by housing an incandescent or halogen bulb in the floor stand and transmitting the light via a built-in fibre optic cable to the operating field. The general surgical field, however, is wider and once the surgeon looks out to this area, it will appear dark, thus the periphery also has to be well-lit with good OR lights.

2.1.2 Theatre equipment

Surgical equipment such as the Operating microscope, the x-ray machine, the coagulation (diathermy) unit, the heart-lung bypass machine and the anaesthetic machines all need to be co-ordinated and well-spaced out (**Figure 1**). In a centre routinely performing these surgeries, there are fixed protocols: they are there for a reason. Surgeons in different centres will do it differently depending on how (and where) they have been trained; therefore, these protocols are to be tailored to the surgeon or institution.

The surgeon's stool (**Figure 1**: inset) is obviously of extreme importance and depending upon their preference should be comfortable and of perfect (adjustable) height with rollers to allow the surgeon to move seamlessly. Different sub-specialties have slightly varying adjustments such back support, arm support (or none) a ring

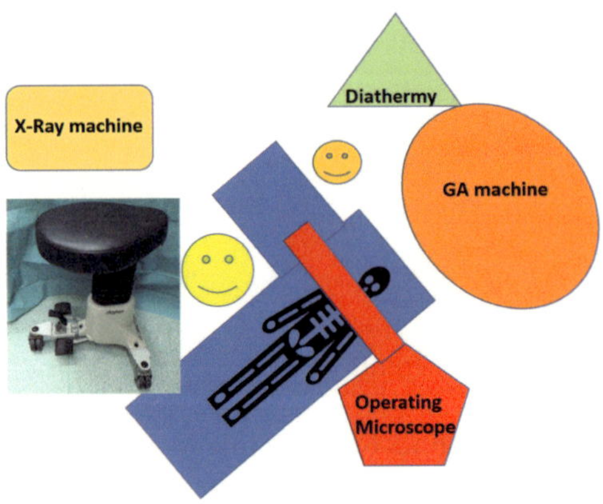

Figure 1.
Operation theatre set-up. The X-ray machine (mini C-arm), operating microscope and diathermy machine should all be away from the main surgeon and not touching the operating table. The surgical stool is shown in the inset.

below to rest the foot and so on. These are personal preferences and every attempt should be made to accommodate them.

The Diathermy cable should be tucked well out of the way and the foot pedal next to the surgeon's dominant foot. If the microscope has foot control, then it could be placed at the assistant's preferred foot or elsewhere. The wire should not interfere with the rollers of the operating surgeon's stool.

2.2 The surgeon

The surgeon performing an operation must be well rested, energised, reasonably hydrated and abreast of the task at hand. It is important to note that any heavy activity (swinging heavy objects, manual activity) should be avoided in the 24 hours prior to microsurgery. If one wants to test this out, try playing table tennis after a round of tennis. Using the larger muscle groups will compromise the fine motor control (in millimetres and micrometres) required in microsurgery. Caffeine intake should be the amount the surgeon is used to: not more and not less. For obvious reasons the use of sedatives prior to surgery is not advised as are medications that may cause drowsiness.

During emergency cases, if progress is not being made, a 10–20-minute break is advised; it usually allows a fresh take on the stumbling block. If it is a technically difficult step, take a breather before starting it, better insight is gained with a few deep breaths.

2.3 The equipment

2.3.1 The operating microscope/loupes

The Operating microscope is used in many different surgical specialities and has been adapted for their particular needs. The Ophthalmic one for example is angled at 45° while the neuro one is used while in standing position. The Plastic and Hand Surgeons use the same one in a sitting position and new the latest ones by Zeiss (Pentero and Kinevo) have 3D images and screens that are facing the surgeon so he does not even have to look down at the field (**Figure 2**)!

The Neuro Microscopes show arterial and venous flow – they also have infrared technology that allows intra-operative visual assessment of blood flow and patency, all with the push of a button.

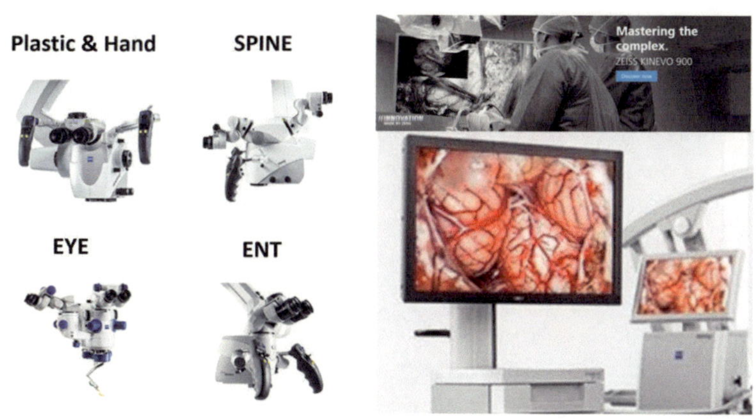

Figure 2.
Operating microscopes. The classic Zeiss microscope came on the S88 floor stand. Now Zeiss has the modern Pentero and Kinevo which can do fluoroscan view as well as show the screen up front (on the right), so the surgeon can operate seeing up, not down, reducing neck strain.

In cases where the vessel diameter is more than 1.5 mm, it is possible to use high powered loupes (4.2x or even 6.0x) to perform the anastomoses safely (by an experienced surgeon). There are now a number of high-quality loupes in the market from various players that provide an extended field of vision with great clarity. It should be noted that the focal length is fixed, so be sure of your working distance before purchasing one.

2.3.2 Surgical instruments

The surgical set for a microvascular anastomosis should be comprehensive (**Figure 3**), however the number of instruments on the table during the repair should be limited to the ones in use and best housed in a silicone-based beaker of water (**not** saline). There are a few essential instruments that one cannot do without: a good microsurgical needle holder, a straight and curved microsurgical scissors, a pair of fine jeweller's forceps (straight and angled) and a vessel dilator [1]. Obviously, it is essential to have a set of microvascular clamps, both single and double, with the latter optional to be mounted on a frame. I prefer the Acland clamps with a bar across (**Figure 4**), which helps to anchor the suture when repairing the vessel. I also like to use a blunt-tipped curved dissecting micro-scissors (**Figure 5**) for it does not damage the adventitial tissue and the all-important intima during vessel preparation.

2.3.3 Sutures

The main suture I use for arterial repair of less than 1.0 mm in diameter is the 10/0 by Ethicon; code W2870 – **Figure 6A**. This has a diameter of 1/1000 of an inch and a length of 13 cm which is one inflexion of the wrist across the operating field under the microscope. There is thus no delay in visualisation i.e. one does not have to move one's vision away from the Operating microscope or drop the needle and pick it up again because the suture is too long. For larger diameter vessels, 9/0 Ethilon may be used or even 8/0 but one has to balance between ease of performance and needle penetration causing leaks. For veins, being thin-walled and more

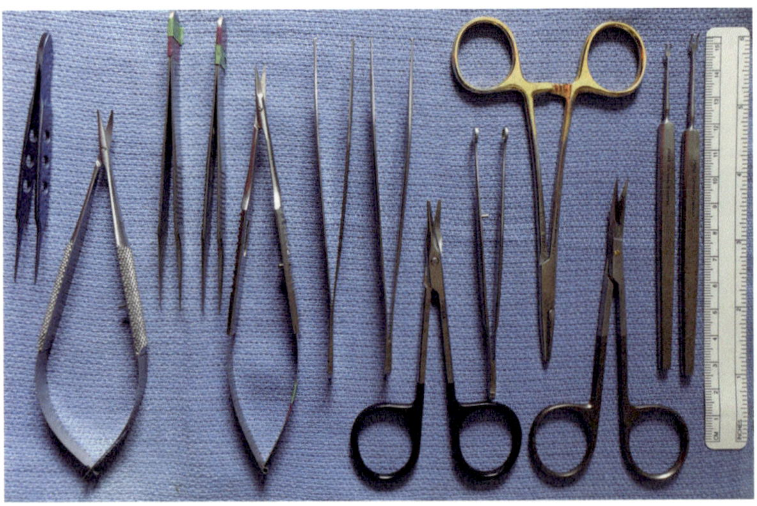

Figure 3.
A basic set of microsurgical instruments. Note the fine double hooks on the right and a nerve holder next to the needle holder. The curved (blunt) micro needle-holder is the second from the left and is extremely useful. The instruments should be comfortable to hold and use.

DOI: http://dx.doi.org/10.5772/intechopen.92903

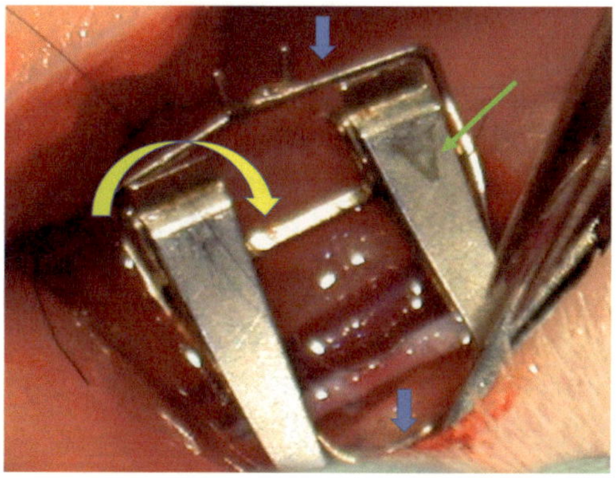

Figure 4.
Double approximator clamps. These thoughtfully designed clamps are mounted on a bar (yellow arrow), where one clamp is fixed whilst the other can slide. Surrounding it is a frame (blue arrows) which assists by allowing one to anchor the suture on to it. The pressure exerted by the clamps (A for artery – green arrow) is approximately 30 g [5, 8].

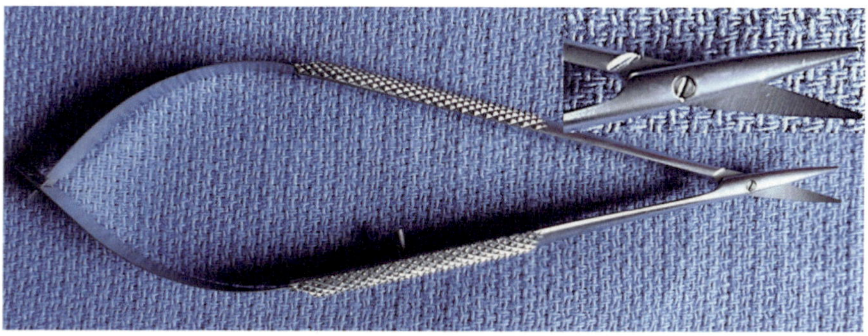

Figure 5.
Blunt tipped micro-scissors (curved). These are excellent for dissecting the soft tissue (adventitia) surrounding the vessels for the blunt tips have less chance of puncturing or damaging the vessel (see magnified inset). Also notice there is hardly a gap when the scissors close (useful feature).

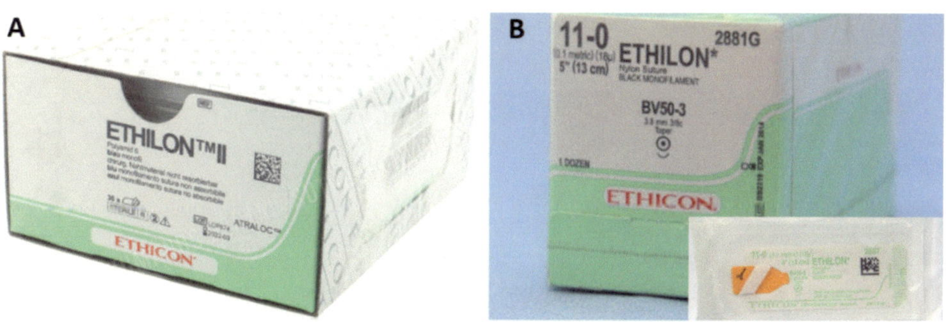

Figure 6.
Ethilon 10/0 and 11/0 sutures from ETHICON. A. The 10/0 suture is 1/1000th of an inch and 13 cm long (W2870, BV75-3 13cm black) B. The 11/0 suture (W2881G, BV50-3 13cm black as in package in inset) is of same length but finer, not visible to the naked eye. These are used at the fingertip for arteries (10/0) and veins (11/0).

challenging to handle, a 10/0 suture is practical. For those more experienced, 11/0 (**Figure 6B**) may be used, although not all theatres carry those. If it is anticipated that the patient's vessels are fragile or small, you may want to forewarn the Sister in charge to obtain the 11/0 sutures.

2.3.4 Other items

Drugs: Syringes of Normal Saline, heparinised saline (1000iu to 50 cc or 100 cc of saline) and Lignocaine 2% are prepared in 10 cc syringes with different coloured cannulas attached to them to differentiate them [3].

Background material (usually made of plastic and blue or green in colour) to place under the anastomosis site during the procedure can be cut to size and prepared. Micro arrowhead sponges to absorb blood and fluids from the surgical site, multiple small single or double skin hooks, white gauze as background around operative field and some folded towels to support one's wrist are all the minute details that will assist in the procedure going smoothly (**Figure** 7).

2.4 The patient

The ideal patient is young and healthy with no co-morbidities, but this is far from reality. For replantation surgery, one must weigh the pros and cons of doing the surgery, for life is more important than limb. Main areas to look out for are cardiac, respiratory, renal, hepatic and clotting functions. In the case of coronary by-pass surgery, obviously life is dependent on the microsurgical aspect, hence the technique must be perfect!

2.4.1 General condition of the patient (e.g. blood pressure)

Several factors affect immediate outcome: the blood pressure (BP) of the patient must be above 110/70 mmHg to ensure good flow through the anastomosed part, a low BP is prone to thrombus formation. Thus, even in a heparinised condition, one has to make sure thrombus formation is not due to inadequate perfusion.

Hypothermia is another cause for failure. One must ensure adequate warmth in the theatre, for the patient as well as the vessel. The anastomosed vessel needs to be kept warm with sterile warm bath or gauze moistened in warm water/saline. We place a bottle of saline in the microwave after unscrewing the cap, and heat it up, then use that. Other modalities include placing a sterile container in a hot water bath to heat up the saline within. Lignocaine 2% can be applied locally to dilate the vessel and reduce spasm after the repair has been completed.

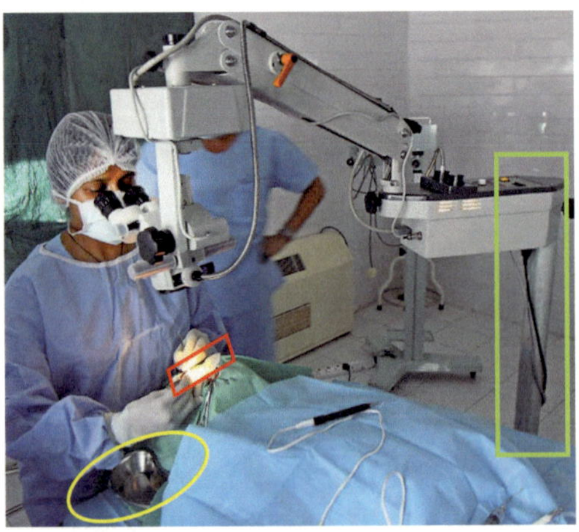

Figure 7.
The operative field. Note the microscope stand (green rectangle) is away from the field allowing the surgeon space to move to the left or right. The right hand should be supported on a roll of towels (yellow oval) and the white gauze (red trapezoid) keeps the background clear (needles visible).

2.4.2 Co-morbidities

The most commonly encountered co-morbidities are Hypertension and Diabetes. The former is not usually an issue, but the latter may well be. Peripheral vascular disease may affect anastomoses in the digital vessels and affect outcome. In central anastomoses, this may not be an issue, but control of the blood sugar level is mandatory in peripheral repair.

When there are multiple co-morbidities, peripheral repair or replantation or even central vascular repair becomes a challenge, not in the technical aspect, but in terms of long-term outcome, due to it being more likely for complications to develop. Where possible, these must be addressed and stabilised **prior to** surgery.

2.4.3 Skin conditions

When there are clues such the red streak sign (**Figure 8**), it means the digit is unfavourable for replantation because of intimal damage and blood leakage. Vein grafting could be attempted but, in the end, it still may fail because there is extensive inner damage.

Severe or dirty abrasion wounds need to be appropriately cleaned or brushed to avoid contamination of the field and delayed infection destroying the repair. Crush injuries cause damage beyond that which is visible and hence should be approached with respect [4].

2.4.4 Operative vessel conditions

If the digital vessel is found in a coiled state or there is a long trailing digital nerve (**Figure 8**), it means this was an avulsion injury (avulsed from the proximal aspect) and the vessel has suffered intimal damage. The entire length requires vein grafting which may leave some areas without a blood supply.

Locally, if there is damage to the vessel ends, these need to be trimmed to a level where they seem intact. On occasion a flap is to be placed for a defect caused by cancer: one must ensure that an irradiated vessel is not used for the anastomosis.

If there is discordance in the size of the donor and recipient vessel, a few tricks are available to harmonise the size mismatch – which needs to be done – to prevent turbulent blood flow [2].

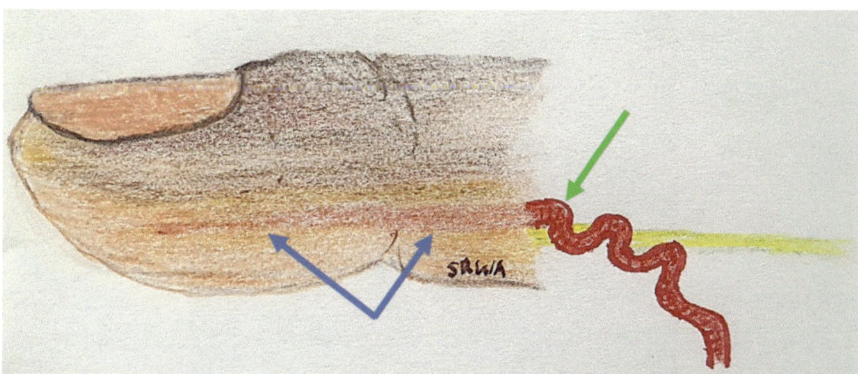

Figure 8.
Red streak sign. The blue arrows point to a faint red line that can be seen where the artery lies. Its intima has been stretched (avulsion injury) and the ecchymosis is due to leakage of blood from avulsed branches. The green arrow shows a red ribbon sign where the vessel is coiled up like a corkscrew due to the avulsion force tearing the layers of the vessel wall. Nerve and tendon may similarly have a long trail. These are poor prognostic signs.

2.4.5 Coagulopathic state

In the medical history it is important to note any features that may give rise to a hypercoagulable state (age, obesity, OCP intake, etc.) and the reverse where a patient is taking anti-coagulants or herbal supplements such as ginseng. In both cases extra steps need to be taken to ensure complications are kept to a minimum.

3. The technique

The initial debridement, dissection and macro fixation (bone, tendon and ligament repair) may be performed under tourniquet control, but the microvascular repair is usually performed without it [3]. The proximal vessel end is clamped (with a single clamp), the tourniquet is deflated (if it was up), and the vessel then tested for good flow by releasing the single clamp. If it has a good **spurt**, the repair is proceeded with. If it does not, the patient is then checked to have good hydration (BP), temperature and oxygenation. Locally, the wound is checked for damage to the proximal vessel or if there is a crush injury [4]. After ruling this out, and ensuring good flow, the proximal vessel end is clamped and flushed with heparinised saline to remove any clots and blood present. Enough length of the vessel is dissected to allow placement in the double clamps, so that a clear view of the end is seen enabling it to be prepared for suturing under magnification. The opposite vessel is similarly prepared and brought into view with the double clamp, making it clearer with a dark coloured background material (**Figure 9**). To achieve these "clear ends", the vessels needs to be "freed" from the surrounding adventitial sheath that they are housed in. I prefer to use the curved dissecting micro scissors (blunt tips) to avoid damaging the vessel wall (**Figure 5**). Care must be taken not to leave any open branches (ligate or clip them) which will cause oozing later. An IV bolus of 1000 U of Heparin is given at this point. I have found this to be enough in the Asian setting. 3000–5000 U causes spontaneous bleeding and I prefer the lower dose.

Once the ends are placed in the clamps, if they are not smooth, they are cut using the adventitial scissors (straight) to provide a sharp clean edge for suturing. It has traditionally been taught to trim the adventitial layer using the sharp adventitia micro scissors, but the blunt-tipped curved micro-scissors allow closer

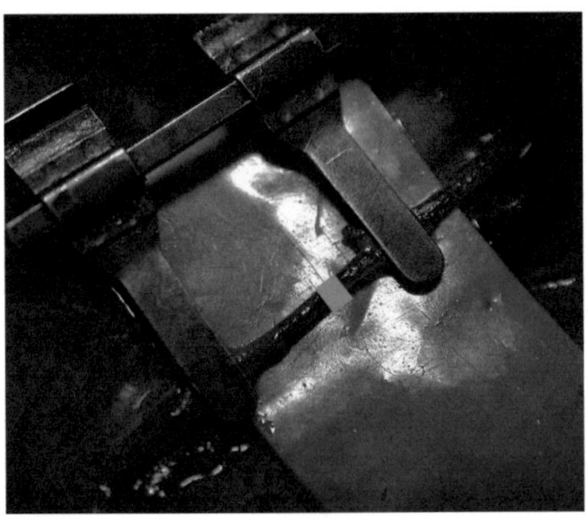

Figure 9.
Placement of vessel ends in double clamps. The two ends of the severed vessel are placed one end in each clamp and brought closer together until they are a vessel diameter apart.

dissection. Hold the vessel by the adventitial layer with the jeweller's forceps and go around the circumference taking off at least 2 mm from the edge (**Figure 10**). Finally, dilate both ends with a fine blunt-tipped vessel dilator to about 1.5 times its original diameter and hold it for 2 seconds [5]. This step is important because not only will it allow better visualisation, it will also stretch the smooth muscle of the intima paralysing it for a couple of hours, so it cannot go into spasm. If there is spasm, 1% or even 2% lignocaine can be applied to the vessel wall to alleviate it. The ends are then rinsed with Heparinised saline and the repair is ready to begin (**Figure 11**).

3.1 Arterial repair: end-to-end

For an end-to-end anastomosis, the vessel ends are usually aligned (and cut if they are prepared vessels) perpendicularly to the vascular axis. If one end is larger than the other, the smaller vessel may be cut at an angle to match the diameter size of the larger vessel (**Figure 12A**).

3.1.1 Triangulation method

In summary, the technique requires the circumference of the vessel wall to be divided into thirds and a stay suture placed at each point (**Figure 12B**). Subsequently sutures are placed between the three stay sutures and depending on the size of the vessel one, two or even three may be squeezed in.

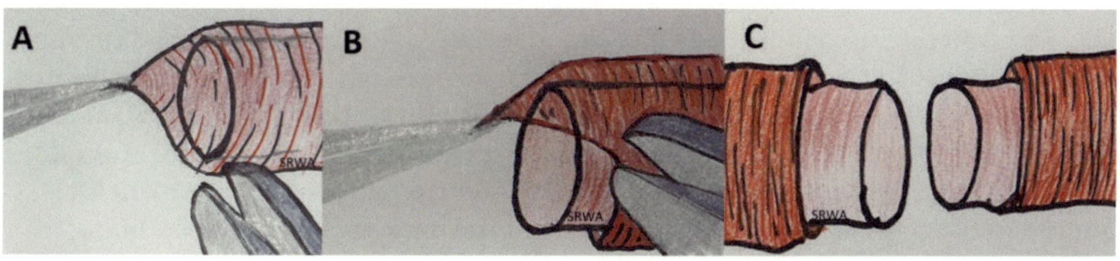

Figure 10.
Trimming the adventitia. (A) The adventitia is pulled using a jeweler's forceps (left hand) and using the micro-scissors (right hand), it is nipped just at the vessel edge (media). (B) With the hole thus created, one blade of the scissors is used to enter, and then cut the adventitia all the way around the vessel, above and below. (C) End result.

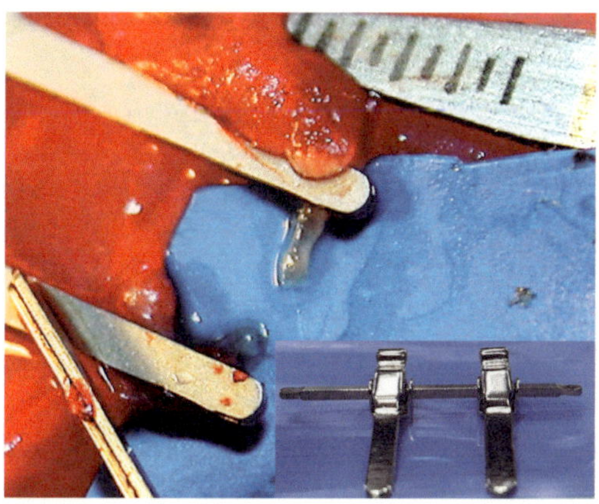

Figure 11.
Prepared vessels. After the adventitia is cleared, the vessels are almost translucent. A dark background and bathing them in saline facilitates repair. Inset: clamps facing the surgeon make certain repair techniques easier.

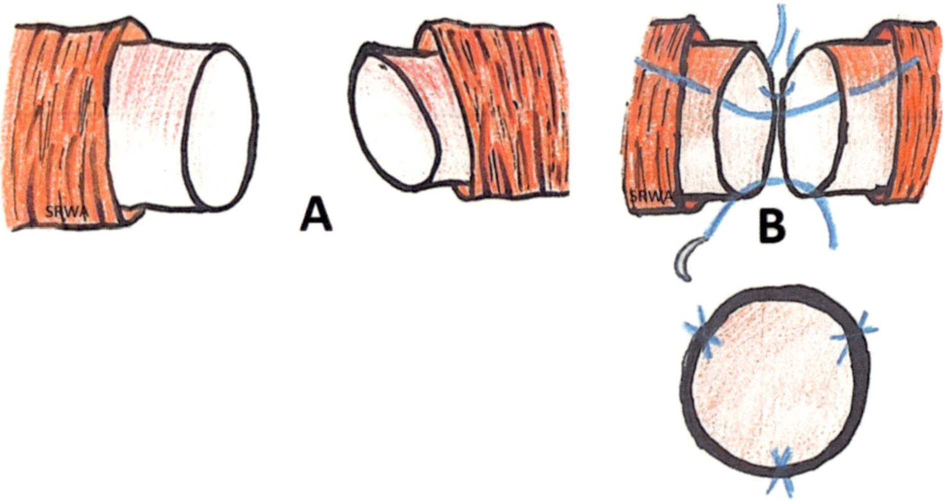

Figure 12.
Triangulation method of repair. (A) If the diameter of the vessel walls are grossly mismatched, the smaller one may be cut obliquely to increase the diameter size. (B) Three stay sutures are placed 120° apart as a guide.

The first stay suture is placed as in **Figure 13**. The needle tip is used to hook the adventitia and the left-hand forceps is placed gently just inside the lumen. The tip of the needle is then pushed into the lumen with the forceps acting as a counterforce [6].

The needle is then brought out and equidistant through the opposite lumen with the left-hand forceps again acting as a resistive force. The needle is pushed through in between the tips of the forceps and picked up in two or three steps gently ensuring the needle swage does not damage the vessel wall and that the thrombogenic cut ends are not inverted inside. Once tied, one thread is kept longer to wind around the clamp bar to stabilise the vessel ends. The first two stay sutures are difficult but especially important because they prevent the back wall of the vessel being caught up. The second suture should be performed in an easy position: on the upper surface of the vessel (**Figure 14**). Once these two are in, two or three intervening sutures are put in. Due to the tightness of the space sometimes it is difficult to place the last two sutures, so it can be modified by not tying the second last suture and continuing the stitching to the last one, leaving the needle in place (**Figure 15**). This allows good visualisation when inserting the needle for the last stitch, preventing catching the 'back wall'. The second last suture is tied followed by the final suture.

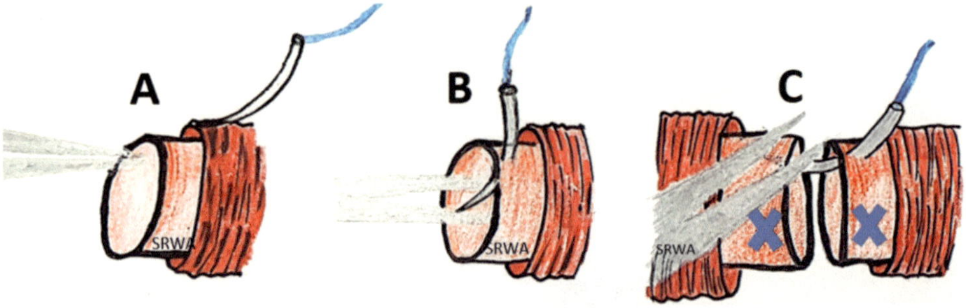

Figure 13.
First stay suture. (A) The adventitial layer is lifted with the tip of the needle and the forceps is gently inserted into the lumen. (B) The needle is then placed on the media and pierced through perpendicularly into the jaws of the forceps tips. (C) A bite on the opposite lumen is similarly placed with the aid of the forceps, this time from outside. × is where the second stay suture should be placed.

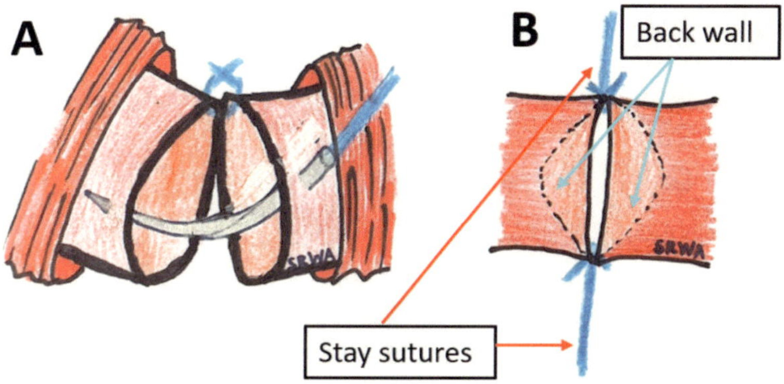

Figure 14.
Second stay suture. (A) The 2nd stay suture is put in at approximately 1/3 of the circumference of the vessel from the first one. It is more difficult to place than the first and is crucial to get it right. Therefore, it is placed in the easier position on the front wall. (B) The two stay sutures are tightened until the front edges approximate in one line.

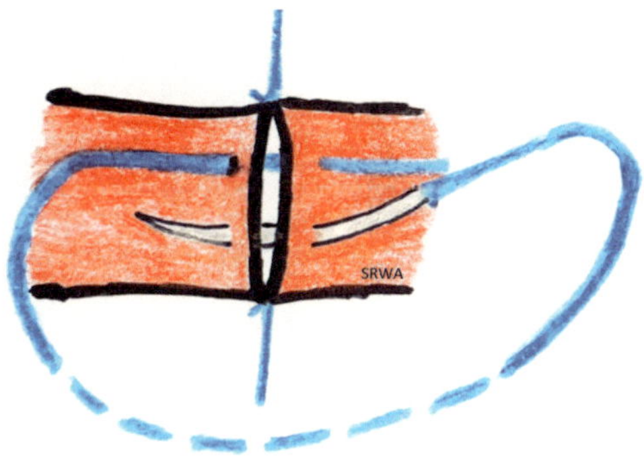

Figure 15.
Double suture. Once the first pass of the needle is done, the knot is not tied and the needle is passed again between the first pass and the last tied suture. The needle is left in situ and the first pass knot is tied by grabbing the free end of the suture. Once this is tied, the needle is pulled through and the second knot tied.

The double clamp may then be flipped 180° and the third suture placed with the back wall up, so it is not taken in with the suturing. The double clamps are moved slightly apart to apply tension on the vessel ends, separating them, allowing the sutured vessel wall to be seen through (**Figure 16**). One can check the repair done as well as safely proceed with the rest of the suturing. The third stay suture is placed equidistant from the other two main stay sutures. The suture is tied and again one end may be wound around the clamp bar to steady the vessel ends. The remaining two thirds of the vessel wall are sutured in a similar fashion. The vessel repair is now complete.

3.1.2 One-way-up

An extremely useful technique to master in situations where there is hardly any manoeuvrability (short vessel length and space) or space to flip the clamp or perform a vascular repair. Suturing is started at the most difficult point in the back wall and done using the inside out technique, moving upwards to easier points.

Place the double clamp with the tips facing you, this will reduce the amount of space they utilise and allow better visualisation (**Figure 11** – inset). Next, place the first suture at the far end of the back wall using the 'inside out' technique so that the knot is outside (**Figure 17A**). The needle is pushed from the outside of the left vessel

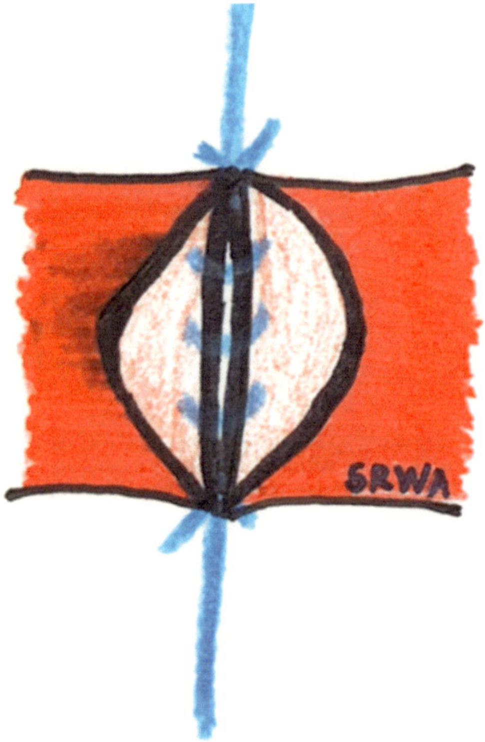

Figure 16.
Doing the back wall. Once the clamps are flipped and tensioned, the view of the sutured first segment can be seen and repair checked before proceeding.

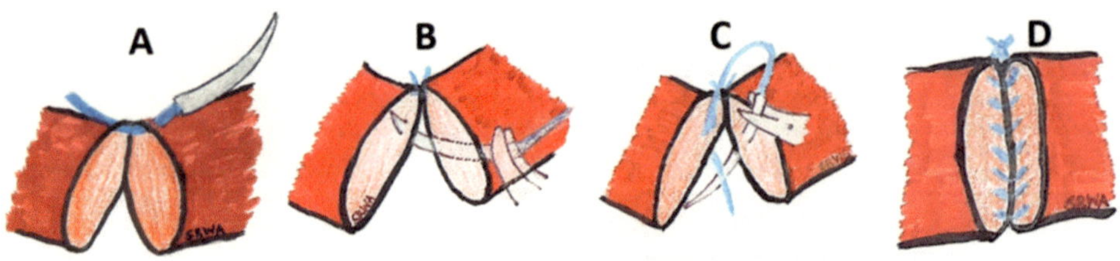

Figure 17.
One-way-up suture technique. (A) Take the first bite the furthest away from you. (B) The second bite is placed next to the first starting with the left vessel wall edge from outside-in. (C) The needle is then pulled out and inserted inside-out of the right vessel wall edge. (D) This is continued to the end till complete.

wall edge to inside the lumen and then it goes from the right vessel wall edge lumen to outside, where the knot is tied. Again, one end is kept long to assist in stabilising the vessel ends. The next suture is placed next to the first one, nearer to you in a similar outside in fashion (**Figure 17B** and **C**), until one moves upwards, then the suturing becomes easier and may be done in the usual way at the top side until complete (**Figure 17D**).

3.1.3 Continuous suturing

In the hands of a practiced surgeon, this suturing technique is rapid and gives good results; however a single mistake may prove costly, requiring the suturing to be redone and perhaps the vessel shortened! Also, a less experienced surgeon may end up entangling the suture or pulling it too tight to cause purse-stringing. Thus, one should only attempt this when one's technique is smooth and well-orchestrated.

In the first few attempts at this technique, the surgeon should aim to divide the vessel end walls into two by putting in one stay suture each on opposing ends. The first stay suture is tied and the long end of the thread is fastened to the clamp bar (**Figure 18**). The opposite is similarly knotted and anchored, but the needled thread is not cut, being used to start the front side of the suturing. Three or maximum four passes with the needle are most likely required in a 1.0–1.5 mm diameter vessel starting with the first one as close as possible to the stay suture to prevent leakage. At the end, any slack in the continuous run is picked up and the suture is tied to the free end of one of the threads. The clamp is then flipped 180° and the needle used to continue suturing the opposing side. Care must be taken not to accidentally take the back-wall for the two are close. Once the other end is reached, the suture is tied to the long thread. The anastomosis is complete.

3.2 Arterial repair: end to side

This technique is an important one to have in the armamentarium. It allows a "way out" for example when there is a paucity of recipient vessels or if the flap donor vessel is too short. It does however carry a risk of size mismatch in terms of diameter and wall thickness. While the former may be somewhat addressed by an oblique cut or narrowing the larger vessel, difference in thickness is more difficult to deal with. The risk of turbulent flow must be born in mind [7].

3.2.1 Preparing the vessel

Ensure the donor vessel is of adequate length to reach the arteriotomy site without undue tension. It must be freed of adventitia at least up to 3 mm away and dilated to ease anastomosis. It is essential to ensure there are no kinks or twists in the donor vessel (artery or especially if it is a vein) because this may be disastrous once it is anastomosed!

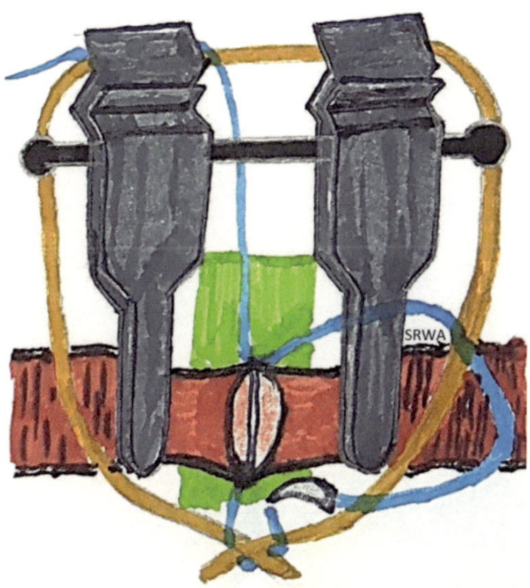

Figure 18.
Continuous suture technique. The vessel is locked by two stay sutures 180° apart. A continuous running suture is started from the distal side proximally.

3.2.2 Making the arteriotomy

Place the artery in double clamps. The arteriotomy site must also be similarly cleared of adventitia to a three times length of the proposed defect. Care should be taken while performing this and instruments must be sharp and well approximated.

A suture is placed at the exact site of the arteriotomy and tied off (**Figure 19A**). It is to be used as an anchor for the excised piece. It is lifted taut and using the left hand, a 45° angled cut is made (**Figure 19B**). The blood is washed out and the micro-scissors are switched to the right hand making a similarly 45° angled cut meeting the opposite side exactly [5].

3.2.3 Technique of suturing

Either one of the three suturing techniques described before (interrupted, one-way-up or continuous) can be used. The key is to start with the right hand on the right-hand side of the arteriotomy and place the suture outside in, then take the donor vessel from inside out (**Figure 19C**). It is a safe practice to place another stay stitch at 180° to stabilise the loose donor vessel. Similarly, a stay stitch mid-distance along on the back wall, can be placed to keep it out of harm's way (**Figure 19D**). The most important point to note in the suturing technique is to angle the stitches radially outwards to the arteriotomy to ensure an even spacing and place them as one would tighten nuts on the wheel of a tyre rim, progress from either side and moving to the centre to complete the anastomosis safely (**Figure 19E** and **F**).

3.3 Releasing the clamps

Once suturing is complete, the clamps are ready to be released but before doing that, make sure the blood pressure is well-maintained, a supply of lignocaine 2%, warm saline, clean gauze and heparinised saline are readily available [8]. Lignocaine is applied to the field and rinsed off with heparinised saline after 2 minutes. The double clamps are approximated, reducing tension on the repair and then the distal

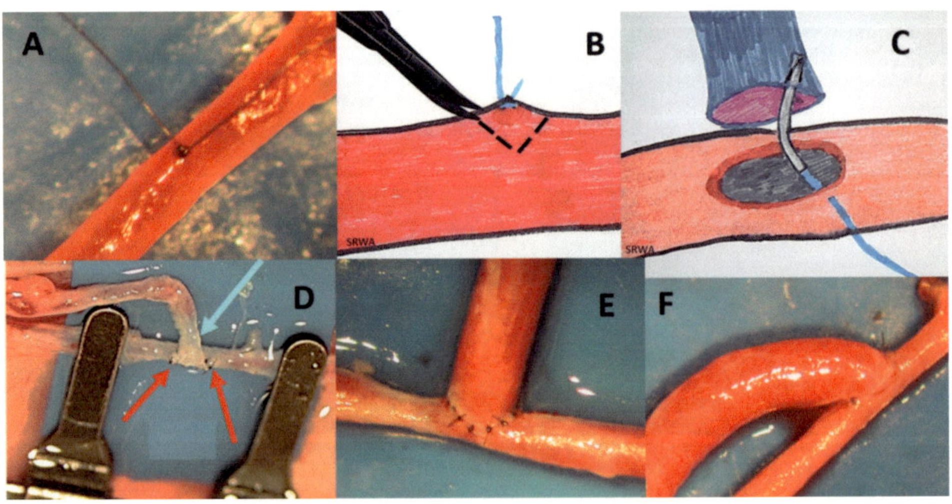

Figure 19.
Performing and end-to-side anastomosis. (A) A suture is tied to the arterial wall (media). (B) A "v"-shaped cut is made. (C) The needle is pushed from the artery to the donor vessel, starting from the right side. (D) Two stay sutures at 180° (red arrows) stabilize the donor vessel; one more is put mid-way at the back (light blue arrow). (E) The sutures are placed radially and evenly. (F) Completed.

one is released first, followed by the proximal one. There will be bleeding, but take the clean gauze, soak it with warm saline and continuously apply light compression on the anastomosis. An infusion of intravenous Heparin is started at this point – I give 4000 U over 24 hours. Previously I would also start the patient on Dextran 40, but now rely on Osmofundin.

After 2 minutes, gently remove the gauze, and rinse with warm saline. If there is no more bleeding, that is good. If there is, you may need to reapply compression and repeat the steps. If it is still spurting, there is a gap which needs closure and this is done with the blood flowing because proximal clamping will result in thrombosis. An assistant provides constant irrigation under which the surgeon performs the suture. If done correctly, it is not difficult but needs intense focus and a steady hand.

3.4 Achieving patency

3.4.1 Evidence of patency

There are a few signs to suggest that the anastomosis is a success. One must learn to appreciate the finer points when trying to decipher the result:

Expansile pulsation means the diameter of the blood vessel increases and decreases with each heartbeat and there is patency of flow. **Longitudinal pulsation** if it is seen proximally, implies the blood is 'hammering' against a block (thrombus) or a wrongly sutured vessel.

Wriggling is movement seen in a curved vessel that is patent and pulsating. It is not observed in straight vessels.

3.4.2 Testing patency

There are several tests that can be performed to illustrate patency and Robert Acland has described them beautifully [5].

The Uplift test shows blood filling and emptying with the systolic and diastolic phases of the heart when an instrument placed under the vessel lifts it up, almost occluding it.

The Empty-and-refill test if done gently provides the most conclusive evidence of patency. A fine curved jeweller's forceps is used to gently occlude the vessel *distal* to the repair. Another pair of forceps is then used to milk the blood in the vessel *distally* and finally the proximal forceps is released (**Figure 20**). If the emptied vessel refills promptly, the repair is patent.

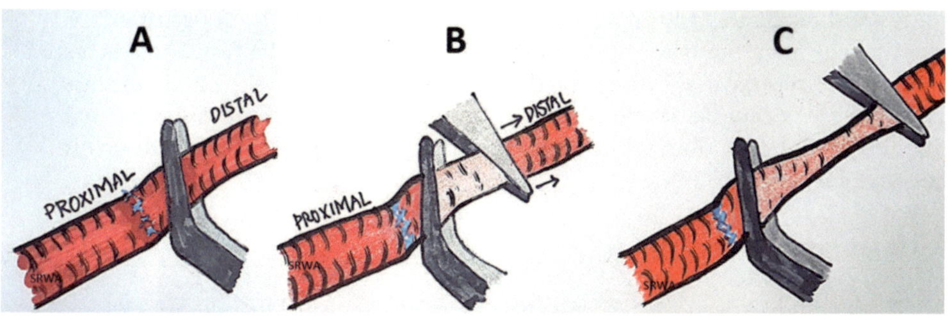

Figure 20.
Empty-and-refill test. (A) An angled forceps is used to hold the vessel distal to the anastomosis. (B) A jeweler's forceps is then used to gently occlude the vessel distal to this. (C) The jeweler's forceps is moved in a distal direction. Upon release of the angled forceps, the vessel will fill up with blood.

3.5 Venous repair: end to end

Repairing a vein is not for the novice and is much harder than an artery. The most obvious reason for this is that the walls are floppy and much thinner, so it is difficult to see the edge after dissection. The other reason is that veins have less adventitial tissue that is rather adherent to its walls, making it challenging to dissect. They are hence also easier to damage unless handled with meticulous care and technique. Last but not least, the slower blood flow makes them prone to thrombosis and even slight damage to the intimal walls kicks off the cascade.

3.5.1 Dissection of the vein

The vascular sheath is flimsy but adherent. Pick it up (making sure one does not damage the venular wall) with a good pair of jeweller's forceps and holding the dissecting (blunt) micro-scissors parallel to the vein, make a hole in it. Then slide the scissors into the space and dissect along the wall of the vein carefully, making sure not to pull out any tributaries with force. These should be ligated with 10/0 nylon or cauterised very carefully. Once released, the vein ends are brought together and placed in the double clamp. The job is made easier if there is an underlying piece of background material and the operative field is flooded with saline or Ringer's lactate. A fine vessel dilator should be used to dilate the vein in two or three directions. It may be difficult to locate the lumen initially, but once this is done, the vein takes a more recognisable form and the lumen becomes visible.

3.5.2 Suturing technique

In view of the thin walls, there is a tendency for the vein edge to roll inwards and mistakes can be made in taking stitches. Extra precaution should be exercised and if there is any doubt, do not proceed until it is cleared. The first two stay sutures are the most crucial and should be done while bathed in saline. The intermediate sutures may be placed slightly further apart (double the distance) than in an artery because venous pressure is lower.

3.5.3 Checking patency

Once the repair is complete, the **distal** clamp is released first to flood the repair site and the vessel dilates immediately. Immediate release of the proximal clamp should show a good flow.

A good result will reveal a similar diameter and colour both proximal and distal to the anastomosis. Patency is confirmed by the uplift test. Flow is tested from distal to proximal (along the direction of flow) across the anastomotic site. If there is a block, it will bulge at the anastomotic site and the proximal diameter will be smaller, while the blood in the distal part will progressively become darker.

3.6 Interpositional vein graft

This procedure is more difficult than a straight-forward venous anastomosis and has multiple steps: getting the arterial defect ready, harvesting a vein for grafting using a meticulous dissection and anastomosing both ends of the graft. It is a necessary skill to acquire for all microsurgeons.

3.6.1 Getting the arterial defect ready

During emergency procedures and sometimes even in elective surgeries, the arterial conduit is damaged and needs replacement in part or more. This is where the interpositional vein graft comes in useful. Most times the vein can be harvested from an adjacent site (size is matched) or a distant one (saphenous in the leg). In all instances, the defect must be measured in order to be bridged. Both the arterial ends are dissected free of adventitia and clamped with single clamps in preparation to receive the vein graft.

3.6.2 Harvesting the vein graft

This is an important step in the procedure and should not be taken lightly. Exact measurement and harvest of the vein graft is to be done by a competent surgeon very carefully. A slightly longer graft is taken in case damage is done to the ends. Too long a graft will cause tortuousness and kinking, while a shorter graft will tend to stretch and tear or leak.

A length of vein corresponding to the arterial defect is outlined (this is measured before the vein is cut) and using the same meticulous dissection techniques described in Section 3.5, the vein graft is extracted after applying clips (or ligating) both ends. Blood is removed from the vein manually and by irrigation. It is placed in the approximator (double) clamp on one side and the anastomosis is ready to begin.

This is started on the right side (for right-handed surgeons) because the artery gives a firm attachment point, and this is needed because the vein graft is free-floating making it difficult to put a suture through. A piece of coloured paper may be used to assist as background material adding oblique cuts to it, so it can help to hold sutures in place while repair is in progress [5].

The second anastomosis is started after the vein graft is checked to avoid any twisting (this will cause kinks and blockages) and that the double clamp is not straddling the repair site.

3.7 Pearls (positive practice)

There are many pearls of wisdom and these are best summarised in tables according to the procedure that is being performed. **Table 1** describes general rules while **Tables 2** and **3** enumerate good practices for arterial and venous repair respectively.

Surgeon	Patient
1. Pre-operative preparation (well-rested, hydration, nutrition and self-relief). 2. Avoid heavy activity the day prior (24 hours). 3. Do not alter (maintain) caffeine intake. 4. Prepare for (elective) surgery mentally.	1. Ensure good hydration. 2. Control of medical conditions (co-morbidities) if any. 3. Peri-operative antibiotics. 4. Review imaging and investigations.
Operation theatre	**Amputated part**
1. Adjust lighting. 2. Maintain OR temperature. 3. Ensure good positioning of machines and instruments. 4. Make sure surgical stool and diathermy foot pedal are in right position. 5. Hands should be well-supported with towels. 6. Place clean gauze as operative field background.	1. Beware of red streak sign. 2. Look for coiled vessels. 3. Look for trailing nerves and tendons. 4. Meticulous pre-dissection. 5. Ensure good spurt of arterial blood.

Table 1.
Pre-operative preparation. This table summarises the various measures the surgeon needs to take prior to starting the surgery to ensure its success.

Positive practice points	Things to avoid
1. Meticulous handling of soft tissues 2. Place (dark) background under vessel ends to see clearly 3. Gentle dissection to skeletonise and isolate vessel 4. Methodical and careful removal of adventitia 5. Rinse blood vessel and dilate it. 6. Approximate clamps	1. Tugging at unyielding tissues. 2. Grabbing the media (full thickness). 3. Performing an action without a clear view or in a pool of blood. 4. Using clamps larger than required. 5. Applying the diathermy to the main vessel.

Table 2.
Tips to achieve a good arterial repair. Points to remember when performing an arterial repair.

Positive practice points
1. Very gentle dissection and minimal handling of vein. 2. Allow the vein to 'rest' after dissection then place it in the clamp. 3. Flush out all the blood, for any standing blood will cause thrombosis. 4. Dilate the vessel with a single prong, then both prongs of the dilator in different directions. 5. After dilation, bathe in lignocaine then apply the clamps. 6. Perform a meticulous anastomosis with evenly placed sutures. 7. Bathe in lignocaine (2–10%) before releasing the clamps. 8. After releasing clamps, allow the blood to flow for a few minutes. 9. If arterial and venous anastomoses are done simultaneously, release the artery clamps just before the vein. 10. If there is a leak, the vein needs to be re-clamped and repaired after the blood is flushed out.

Table 3.
Tips to achieve a good venous repair. Veins need more care in their handling and rest periods in between steps. A keen eye will prevent mishaps such as catching the back wall inadvertently.

3.8 Pitfalls (negative practice)

While there are an enormous number of things that can go wrong with even the most experienced surgeon, I have tried to list the most common ones here in order as they appear in the text: Various arterial repair techniques of increasing difficulty (**Tables 4** and 5), venous anastomosis (**Table 6**) and grafting (**Table** 7) and finally arteriotomy and end-to-side repair (**Table 8**).

Positive practice points	Negative actions to avoid
1. Have a clear operative field of vision and good access 2. Mobilise a good length of vessel 3. Properly trimmed adventitia and clean vessel ends 4. Comfortable spacing of clamps 5. Divide the vessel into equal thirds and place sutures equidistant from both vessel ends. 6. Clear view and sure of needle placement.	1. small and inadequate wound, poor retraction leading to poor visualisation 2. Trying the anastomosis with short vessel ends 3. Persisting in the anastomosis when view is obstructed or when facing trouble. 4. Excessive traction (clamps too far apart) or obscured view of lumen (clamps too close). 5. Asymmetrical placement of sutures with bad coaptation of vessel ends 6. Struggling with needle then catching the back wall.

Table 4.
Arterial repair technique: Triangulation. The column on the left lists the positive actions to be practiced while the column on the right, the negative results thereof.

One-way-up technique
1. Have the tips of the clamps facing you. 2. Make the first stitch furthest away from you 3. Start with the difficult side first and place sutures on either side of the first stitch 4. Avoid entangling your suture when placing the second half of the stitch 5. Work your way up carefully
Continuous suture technique
6. Divide the vessel ends into equal halves 7. Do not use too long a suture to prevent entanglement 8. Keep the stitches evenly placed and pull the thread to evenly tighten it at the end 9. Make sure the knots are squarely tied and secure.

Table 5.
Pointers in performing arterial repair. Tips to ensure good results in the two other (more challenging) techniques of arterial repair.

1. Aggressive dissection and 2. Incorrect handling of the vein with forceps, scissors or bipolar coagulator. 3. Frequent picking up and letting go of the vessel wall. 4. Suturing inverted vessel edges. 5. Picking up the back wall.

Table 6.
Pitfalls in venous anastomoses. These are the common mistakes made when anastomosing veins. Extra care needs to be taken in handling them because they tend to thrombose easily.

Pearls	Pitfalls
1. Ensure right diameter of the vein graft 2. Measure the length of graft **before** harvesting. 3. Take the vein graft with a cuff of fat around it. 4. Lay the vein graft straightened out (untwisted) with both sides in clamps. This avoids twisting with no blood in graft, while ensuring its visibility. 5. Remember to reverse the vein graft for arterial flow to accommodate for the valves.	1. Suturing two vessels of mismatched diameters 2. The vein graft shortens after harvest! 3. A skeletonised graft is more susceptible to damage by the forceps. 4. Not checking for a twist before the second anastomosis may result in unnecessary anguish! 5. Using suction while graft is in the operative field is dangerous! Clamps also help avoid it being sucked in. 6. Getting the clamps in the way of the anastomoses may necessitate redoing it!

Table 7.
Pearls and pitfalls of vein graft harvest and anastomosis. Performing the right steps in the correct order not only increases chances of success but also reduces time and effort taken.

1. Perform the arteriotomy in the steps mentioned in the text. 2. Angle the adventitia scissors at 45° to make the cut. 3. Remember to reverse the vein graft and place it straightened out (while still in the clamps). 4. Start with the arterial wall from outside in and take the vein inside out. 5. Place a second stitch at 180° to the first. 6. Place the sutures radially spaced and not longitudinal to the arteriotomy 7. Put in a stay suture on the back wall mid-way between these first two stitches. 8. Any technique may be used to perform the anastomosis. 9. Keep a short leash on the suture length 10. If using continuous suturing, tighten as you move along.

Table 8.
Perfecting end-to-side repair. Pointers to bear in mind when performing this in addition to what has been mentioned earlier.

4. Conclusion

In conclusion, microsurgical anastomosis is a fine art that needs practice, practice, practice to make perfection. There is absolutely no room for error. There are numerous techniques that can help the novice, though and repetition will improve the outcome. Good instrumentation, the correct suture materials and an excellent microscope will help tremendously. A number of items may be modified without sacrificing the result and some of these ideas may be used in less developed countries.

Acknowledgements

I would like to thank Intechopen for their generosity in helping with the funding of this chapter.

Conflict of interest

There is no conflict of interest to be declared.

Author details

Sharifah Ahmad Roohi
Hand and Upper Limb Centre, Pantai Hospital, Kuala Lumpur, Malaysia

*Address all correspondence to: roohihandsurgery@gmail.com

References

[1] Cobbett JR. Microvascular surgery. In: Birnstingl M, editor. Peripheral Vascular Surgery: Tutorials in Postgraduate Medicine. Vol. 3. London: William Heinemann Medical Books Ltd; 1973. Ch. 17. pp. 384-391

[2] Rahman MN, Shahriman AB, Za'aba SK, Roohi SA, WAN K, Ayob MN, et al. Computational fluid dynamic analysis of the effect of kink conduit in microvascular vein grafting. International Journal of Mechanical and Mechatronics Engineering (IJMME). 2012;**12**(6):53-59

[3] Godfrey AM, Lister GD, Kleinert HE. In: Birch R, Brooks OM, editors. The Hand 4th ed. (Rob and Smith's Operative Surgery). London: Butterworths; 1998. pp. 85-91

[4] Roohi SA, RWH P. Crush injuries of the hand part II: Clinical assessment, management and outcomes. In: Salgado AA, editor. Essentials of Hand Surgery, First on Line Edition. Mexico City: InTechOpen; 2018. DOI: 10.5772/intechopen.78298

[5] Acland RD, Sabapathy SR. Acland's Practice Manual for Microvascular Surgery. 3rd ed. Mumbai, India: Indian Society for Surgery of the Hand; 2008

[6] Butler CE, Adelman DM. Principles of microsurgery. In: Thorne CH et al., editors. Grabb's Plastic Surgery. 7th ed. Philadelphia: Lippincott Williams & Wilkins; 2014

[7] Lee HL, Shahriman AB, Yaacob S, Zuradzman MR, Khairunizam WAN, Zunaidi IB, et al. In vitro evaluation of finger's hemodynamics for vein graft surveillance using electrical bio-impedance method. Australian Journal of Basic and Applied Sciences. 2014;**8**(4):350-359

[8] Richard M, Lewis GJ, Levin S. In: Hunt TR III, Wiesel SW, editors. Operative Techniques in Hand Wrist and Forearm Surgery. Philadelphia: Lippincott Williams & Wilkins; 2011. pp. 796-807